WHAT OTHERS ARE SAYING...

Wonderful book! It poignantly describes the trials and tribulations of coping with a loved one with a disease that insidiously tears apart the very fabric that makes us human. I am confident this book will be of comfort to caregivers as well as anyone with a friend or loved one with Alzheimer's disease.

Lawrence Weinberg, MPH, MD
Neurology

It is rare to find a book on this subject that probes, as this does, the range and depth of emotions experienced by caregivers of Alzheimer's victims. This pioneering book should encourage other caregivers to publicly share rather than hide their own personal trauma. The author's frank and sometimes graphic account of her journey with her father enables us to gain a clearer picture of the tragedies and triumphs of such a journey.

Lew Jurey, Aerospace Engineering Consultant
and friend

"Where's my shoes?" is an uplifting book written with honesty and humor. Not only is it a must read for families and caregivers who deal with this insidious disease day-to-day and hour-by-hour, but it's also an inspiring journal that helps all of us better understand the debilitating effects of Alzheimer's and the tribulations family members face.

Lois Erisey Poole, Author and
Syndicated Columnist

"Where's my shoes?" captures the roller coaster ride that is Alzheimer's...a must read for anyone exploring the peaks and valleys of how one family deals with this debilitating disease.

Roberta Widmer, Administrator
VNA Adult Day Care

...a poignant account of a daughter thrust into the role of caregiver; her fears, uncertainties, and resolution of situations not bargained for in her role in life. *"Where's my shoes?"* exposes the reader to the range of emotions that all caregivers go through.

Ken and Sally Howard
The author's "adopted" parents

Brenda shows the effect Alzheimer's can have on the affected person, on the caregiver, and on the entire family. Brenda's experience reveals the difficult choices our loved ones may one day have to make for each of us. As Brenda's husband, I could not believe all that we accomplished, learned, and faced together in dealing with her father's disease. This book is a must for anyone contemplating caring for a person with Alzheimer's or for anyone who is already a caregiver.

David Borden
The author's husband

A timely, sometimes funny, informative story of one family's journey.
J. Parsons, Retired Nurse
Caretaker to her 86-year old mom with Alzheimer's

Martin reminds me of my father who passed away a few years back. *"Where's my shoes?"* was very touching and I shed a few tears while reading it. I was reminded that we're often stronger than we think. It renewed my courage and gave me the strength to do more.

Jan Ferguson
The Barefoot Lady

A loving daughter's sad but heartfelt memories and day-by-day experiences of her dad's decline from the debilitation of Alzheimer's disease. A most helpful aid for ALL caring caregivers, and a *must* read for all students in training.
Marlys Meckler, Speech Pathologist
Director, Tarzana Speech and Language Center
Team Member, Center for Aging Research and Evaluation

As the daughter of a father with Alzheimer's, I found that Ms. Avadian so aptly describes incident after incident that challenge caregivers to their limits. Her book details how this disease so tragically robs its victims of every human dignity.

Katie Corbett
Newspaper Journalist and Editor

Had Ms. Avadian's book been available during the six years I cared for my wife with Alzheimer's prior to her placement in a nursing facility, I could have saved myself many heartaches and much aggravation. Ms. Avadian's literary style, blending pathos, humor and philosophy is just the icing on the cake and makes fascinating reading for anyone.

Jonathan Schulkin
Appreciative Caregiver

As a professional who spends many hours...trying to help caregivers of dementia patients solve some of their problems, I continue to be amazed at their strength, patience, and humor. This book personifies what I see and allows the reader to become a member of this family for a short while. This is a must read for caregivers and professionals.

Marlene V. Harrison, RN-C, BS
Program Director for the Center for
Aging Research and Evaluation
Granada Hills Community Hospital

This book imparts visions and memories both poignant and pleasurable of my beloved husband who has Alzheimer's.

Patti Compton
Caregiver to the Love of Her Life

One of the most memorable lectures I heard was by the Base Chaplain prior to our departure for Air Force Survival Training in July, 1961. I had just completed pilot training and was about to enter a grueling three-week survival experience constantly pursued by aggressor forces, covering many miles each day in the Northern California mountains, while living completely off the land.

The lecture was entitled, "I Will Lift Up Mine Eyes Unto the Hills" and is excerpted here.

> "As you embark upon this challenge, all of you will have many varied experiences, but I can tell you with certainty that all of you will have one common experience. Sometime during this trek you will meet someone face-to-face, you will not be able to ignore him. You may like him or you may despise him but you will meet him. I can even tell you when each of you will meet him. It will be when you are starving, totally exhausted, cold, wet, and scared. It is then when you will be staring directly into his face. This person will be YOU! You will not have seen yourself before like this. Ask him, 'Do you have the commitment to see this through to its conclusion? Are you going to give up?' Reach into yourself and find the strength to continue. Make sure to come to like this person."

Brenda came face-to-face with this person many times as chronicled in *"Where's my Shoes?"*. Her trek was exhausting, filled with unknowns and hazards. She found the strength to keep going, to see this through.

Dave ("Ferg") Ferguson
Combat Pilot—two tours in Vietnam and
Flight Test Pilot—first to fly the YF-22

"Where's my shoes?"

My Father's Walk Through Alzheimer's

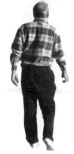

More than a book *about* Alzheimer's, the author openly reveals details about *caring* for someone with dementia.

BRENDA AVADIAN, M.A.

North Star Books
Lancaster, California

Copyright © 1999 by Brenda Avadian

Published by NORTH STAR BOOKS
P.O. Box 259
Lancaster, California 93584-0259

Publisher's Cataloging-in-Publication Data
Avadian, Brenda.
    "Where's my shoes?": my father's walk through Alzheimer's / Brenda
    Avadian – Lancaster, Calif.: North Star Books, 1999.
        p.   cm.
    Includes index and bibliography.
    ISBN 0-9632752-1-6
        1. Alzheimer's disease—Patients—Care. 2. Alzheimer's disease—
        Patients—Biography. 3. Avadian, Martin. I. Title.
RC523.2.A923 A93   1999   98-87480
362.1'96831'0092   dc—21   CIP

PROJECT COORDINATION BY JENKINS GROUP, INC.

02 01 00 99 ◆   5 4 3 2 1

Printed in the United States of America

Photo Credits and Captions:
Front cover: Photographer: Brenda Avadian. Model: Lew Jurey.
Back flap: Martin and Brenda Avadian, Milwaukee, 1996. Photographer: David J. Borden.
Page 207: Martin Avadian at Catalina Island, March 1997. Photographer: Lew Jurey.

Dedicated to my father,
Martin Avadian,
*who taught me the value of perseverance
and with whom I share a birthday.*

And to all caregivers.

"Where's my shoes?" was written to increase care-givers' insights and awareness of options—and to reduce the feelings of loneliness that can overwhelm all caregivers.

According to the Alzheimer's Association, over four million people in the United States alone suffer from Alzheimer's. Ten percent of people aged sixty-five and older have Alzheimer's, while fifty percent of people aged eighty-five and older are afflicted.

To assist in the care of those with Alzheimer's, the proceeds from this book's sale will be donated directly to individuals, groups, and organizations who help people with Alzheimer's and their caregivers.

CONTENTS

FOREWORD

*H*OW-TO BOOKS FOR CAREGIVERS OF PEOPLE WITH ALZHEIMER'S disease have been published and dryly cloned for mass consumption over the past twenty years since Alzheimer's hit the public spotlight. A uniquely personal touch is what sets this book apart from the pack.

The author gives us significant insight into her family dynamics and personal struggles in managing her father's declining health, while maintaining his dignity and her own sense of self.

The shoes become a metaphor and focal point of expression for waning independence and autonomy on the one hand and an attempt to control unacceptable behavior on the other. This battle takes on such dramatic proportions that it provides an unexpected source of comic relief as the household ends up hiding the shoes from each other and the aging fox temporarily out-maneuvers the younger hounds.

This tender book encompasses much more than a family's confrontation with Alzheimer's disease, though it provides useful information for others who are traveling down this dreadful road. Ms. Avadian manages to paint a portrait of Americana through the reflection of her immigrant father's life who, through honesty and hard work, made his Midwestern American dream come true for himself and his family.

His quiet, understated, and generally under-recognized efforts are captured and shared in this book and serve as a loving tribute to him. An emotional and paradoxical moment occurs near the end of the book when he is given a chance to read and savor excerpts of the pre-published manuscript through the dimming eyes of his cognizance.

This book should find broad appeal among family members who are struggling with this disease and with those who seek meaning through the lives of their forefathers and mothers who helped pave their way.

ROLAND JACOBS, M.D.
DIPLOMATE, AMERICAN BOARD OF PSYCHIATRY AND NEUROLOGY
ADDED QUALIFICATIONS IN GERIATRIC PSYCHIATRY

PREFACE

*T*HIS BOOK WAS INSPIRED BY MY FATHER WHO WAS DIAGNOSED WITH dementia of the Alzheimer's type. After becoming his caregiver, I began a journey that would have a major effect upon my life. It is said that if we learn from life's experiences, we will grow. I was unprepared for how much I was to grow.

As the days progressed into weeks and the weeks into months, I put aside my life and career in order to care for my father. I formed timeless relationships and bonds with people who also cared for their loved ones with Alzheimer's. These relationships formed the fabric of my life and reduced my feelings of isolation and loneliness.

As the disease took its toll on my father, I suffered great pain and learned new things. To make sense of the highs, the lows, the uncertainties and the inexplicable, I kept a private journal. This journal contains my joy and my agony.

After encouragement from caregivers and professionals, I set aside time to write this book—as a tribute to my father while he is still alive—and as a source of guidance for you, the caregiver.

By sharing my heartfelt experiences with you, I hope you will feel united with people who have and will join you on your journey down the road of your loved one's Alzheimer's. I also hope you will gain some knowledge by reading these pages—and comfort from knowing that you are not alone.

Although we may not know each other personally, and may never have the good fortune to meet, we are joined by our common experience.

I wish to give something back to the people who have cared for my father, and to help others. Therefore, I am donating the proceeds from the sale of this book to individuals, groups, and organizations who help people with Alzheimer's and their families.

ACKNOWLEDGMENTS

As with any worthy endeavor, many people contributed to this book.

The following reviewers (listed alphabetically) were the first to review this book: Patti Compton, Katie Corbett, Lois Erisey Poole, Dave and Jan Ferguson, Sally and Ken Howard, Jeanne Parsons, Jonathan Schulkin, and Roberta Widmer. Special thanks to Lois, who not only marked all but seven pages in the original manuscript but sat down with me for several hours to discuss her comments in detail. Lois also encouraged me to include the "Ten Suggestions" section at the end of this book.

Thank you to the caregivers who got our "Ten Suggestions" list started by being the first to submit theirs: Pat Adams, Patti Compton, Paul F. Harmon, Helen Jones, Marina McCarthy, and Jonathan Schulkin.

Special thanks to the VNA's Adult Day Care Support Group in the Antelope Valley, whose feedback I regularly sought throughout the development of this book.

Special thanks to the members of the North Los Angeles County Women Writer's Network, who proposed the title of this book and whose continuing suggestions were always welcome.

Special thanks to Reuben Cano and Steve Masser, who designed our Internet websites in order to help caregivers become aware of this book.

Special thanks to the Granada Hills Community Hospital's Center for Aging Research and Evaluation, for their advice and support during the final stage of this book.

Special thanks to Joel Roberts, whose *Excellence in Media* workshop in Beverly Hills gave me the voice with which to share my heartfelt thoughts.

Thank you to the following people (listed alphabetically) who took time from their busy schedules to give me welcome advice: Lou Bozigian, Ann Harris, Betty Klingkamer, and Bill Multanen.

A special thank you to Lew Jurey, who gave up his sleeping and weekend hours to edit the manuscript and to advise me about the cover, photography, and layout. Lew also modeled for the cover photo.

Thank you to the team at the Jenkins Group, who coordinated the prepress (Jerrold Jenkins, Susan Howard, Theresa Nelson, Alex Moore, and Nikki Stahl). A special thank you to Mary Jo Zazueta, editor extraordinaire, who must have used more than one red pencil on this manuscript and whose designing prowess gives this book its warmth and appeal. Also, a special thank you to Eric Norton, whose cover design honors the words inside and conveys my heartfelt passion for this book.

Special thanks to Jack Canfield, Mark Victor Hansen, Dan Poynter, and Dottie Walters, whose ideas during the *How to Build Your Speaking & Writing Empire* workshop, further fueled my passion and gave me a map to follow.

Finally, a very special thank you to David Borden, my husband and partner for twenty-one years, without whom I could not have taken this caregiving journey nor completed this book.

WARNING-DISCLAIMER

This book was written to help caregivers gain greater awareness of caring for someone. It is sold with the understanding that the publisher and author are not engaged in rendering legal or other professional advice. If legal or other expert assistance is required, the reader should seek the services of a competent professional.

It is not the purpose of this book to provide all the information available about Alzheimer's—rather it is to offer the reader as accurate a description as possible of the details that unfolded in one family's experience with Alzheimer's.

People's names were included in the book with permission. Since this book was written and published to help other caregivers, both positive and negative experiences are included. Where experiences were unfavorable, permissions were not sought nor were the parties' names included. The purpose of this book is not to damage a reputation but rather to present a realistic account of the events that unfolded.

The author and North Star Books shall have neither liability nor responsibility to any person and/or entity with respect to any loss or damage caused, or alleged to be caused, directly or indirectly by the information contained in this book.

If you do not wish to be bound by the above, you may return this book (in resalable condition) to the publisher for a refund.

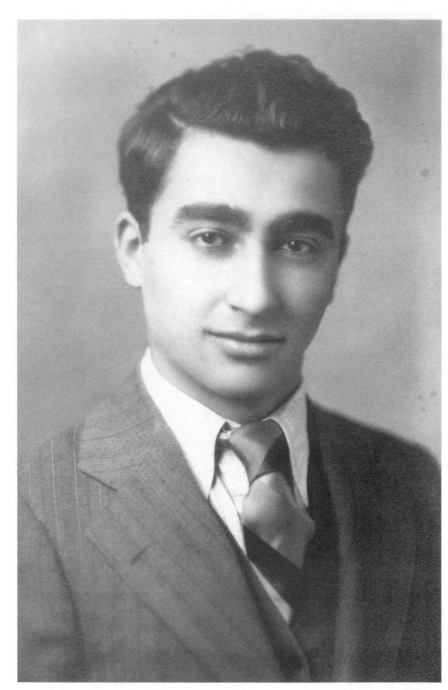

Martin Avadian at eighteen. Chicago.

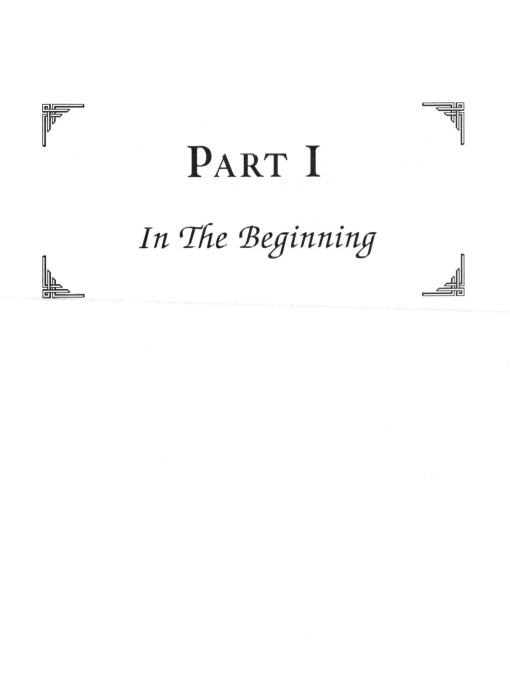

PART I

In The Beginning

My father has lived through the most dynamic period in history. He lived through two world wars, the Korean War, Vietnam, and Desert Storm. Although he is fiercely patriotic, he was too young to serve in World War I and too old for World War II. He has witnessed massive technological changes during his eighty-eight years on this earth, from the Spirit of St. Louis to Neil Armstrong walking on the moon; from handwritten letters mailed with two-cent stamps to virtually free electronic mail arriving across the world in seconds!

Born in 1910 in Van, Armenia, Martin Avadian was eight years old when his father was declared missing in action during the Armenian genocide. Two years later, he and his mother sailed to the United States, where they settled in Chicago with his mother's sister. His mother soon remarried.

Martin was a diligent student and tried to learn everything. He wanted to continue going to school, but money was scarce and he didn't want to take advantage of his stepfather. So he began his independence by working odd jobs, doing anything a young teenager could to earn money.

Martin was a hard worker. After years of working jobs for meager wages, he was hired as a machinist at General Electric. He saved money at a feverish rate. His investment strategy was conservative yet consistent. During the 1950s, earning $100-plus a week, he withdrew $10 from every check to buy U.S. Savings Bonds. He also accumulated General Electric stock over the years. With the increase in the stock market, his shares appreciated over $100,000 in less than one year. His attorneys and accountant asked, "How could a machinist accumulate so much?"

A long-time bachelor, he married at the age of thirty-nine, started a family, and bought a house (with a $3,000 loan from his mother which he paid back in only two weeks).

My father was a private man. While growing up, I used to gaze at his high school graduation picture in a gray, wooden frame that sat untouched on the mantelpiece. I imagined what kind of person he was more than thirty years before I came into the world. Looking through his files I found pictures of a handsome gentleman, 5'6" tall and 145 pounds, who prided himself on his stylish clothing and immaculate grooming. The years that followed, spanning almost a half-century, would take away much of his hearing and shrink his body to a meager 5'1" and 118 pounds.

Chapter 1

HOW IT ALL BEGAN

*M*Y HUSBAND AND I MOVED TO CALIFORNIA in 1989, about 1,800 miles away from our hometown in Wisconsin. My parents still lived in Wisconsin; so we flew back every year to visit. Our annual visits enabled us to recapture the years of our youth, when we Midwesterners had big plans to achieve mighty dreams. These trips gave us Californians (albeit neophyte Californians) the opportunity to return home to see our family and friends.

As circumstances changed, we began to visit Wisconsin more frequently—every six months or so.

My mother had an enlarged heart. It was so weak it couldn't efficiently pump enough blood to prevent her lungs from drowning. My brother and sister were frequently called to rush her to the hospital. Ma would gasp for air as they raced through traffic, violating traffic lights trying to reach the hospital before she took her last breath. (My mother hated the noise and commotion of ambulances so my sister, who lived five blocks away, and my brother, who lived with my parents, became her emergency transportation service.) Ma was close to death so many times, my husband and I would return to spend time with her, thinking, "This will be the last time we'll see her alive."

My mother always had a strong influence over us. She was best described by others as having an uncanny resemblance to Mother Teresa. Her petite and frail appearance defied her strong will. She modeled the ideals of hard work and perseverance.

After valiantly fighting for her life for over a decade, she died in Milwaukee on April 1, 1993.

My father called me with the news. I couldn't believe it! She left us on, of all days, April Fools' Day! The conversation with my father went something like this:

"Brenda, how are you? I hope I'm not interrupting anything. I'm calling to let you know Ma died."

First, my father never called me—too expensive to talk long distance, so I called him every month. Second, was he kidding? This is strange, my father calling me on April Fools' Day. I decided not to be a victim of his joke.

I exclaimed, "You've got to be kidding!"

"No," came his serious and somber reply.

"C'mon, it's April Fools'. Whad'ya tryin' to pull?"

My father replied, "I couldn't believe it myself when the nurse called only one hour after I had left her!"

I kept track of my mother's progress by calling her at home and at the hospital when she was in intensive care. The nurses would hold the phone to her ear while we talked. So I was quite surprised when I called the Intensive Care Unit and the nurse explained that Ma had checked out nearly two weeks ago! I asked if she had been transferred to another area of the hospital, and she said, "No." The nurse explained that the doctor said there was nothing more they could do for Ma. My first thought was she died, and no one had told me! I learned later that Ma had been placed in a twenty-four-hour skilled nursing facility.

My father continued, "In fact, I thought the nurse was kidding me and I told her so! But she assured me that when she came back into Ma's room Ma had passed away."

"Wow," was my reply. *Did I feel like a fool!* "Mardig, how are you doing?"

"Well, under the circumstances, I'm doing all right. I'm just a bit surprised!" *My father, the diplomat, the gentleman, and master of controlling his emotions.*

"Well, I'll come back then. What do you need?" I asked.

"Oh no, don't come. You're working. Don't take off time from work."

My father worked at General Electric for thirty-two years without missing one day of work. He received special recognition for this rare achievement.

"Mardig, *(We called my father by his first name, Martin, which loosely translated to Armenian, is Mardig.)* I will come. This is not a decision for you to make. I will help you with Ma. Besides, our family must be together during this time."

"No, that is not necessary. I have taken care of everything."

"Oh yeah? What have you done?"

We went around and around, quarreling, after which he finally agreed to let me return to help him and to spend time with him. It turned out he had not made all the preparations.

A day or two later, David, my husband, flew back and joined me, and we helped Mardig make arrangements. We tried to make this a family event by getting my sister and brother involved—to no avail. So, it was up to Mardig, David, and me to do the best we could for my mother, including her wish to be cremated. Even though Mardig had already purchased a niche for both of them, he wanted his wife's cremains (ashes after cremation) at home for a while.

David and I thought it would be a good idea to have a family gathering where we'd scatter some of her cremains under the two trees she had planted and tenderly cared for before her death. It was not to be. No funeral, no family gathering, nothing. Neither my sister nor brother showed up during the entire time David and I were there. My father was disappointed, but he did not dwell upon it.

We would not be deterred. David and I spent a lot of time with Mardig and listened to him tell stories about his life and the places he'd like to visit. With his conditional acceptance, we even planned a multi-country trip for October. We planned to visit Armenia (Mardig's birthplace), Moscow (all of us wanted to see this city), and Germany (to enjoy the beer during Oktoberfest). Although Mardig didn't drink alcohol, he held a longtime fascination with Germany. David and I, on the other hand, enjoy great beer!

As the time drew near for us to depart upon this adventure, it became more apparent that Mardig was not prepared to take the trip. There was nothing seriously wrong to prevent him from doing so. In fact, he was healthier and in better shape than I was at forty-nine years his junior! No, it was something much more regrettable. It was all of the excuses he made; excuses we all make.

"Oh, I have so much to do. I have Ma's bills to pay. They're still coming, you know. I have to straighten out the house. There's papers everywhere that need to be organized. I still have to pay taxes. The basement is a mess. I have tools laid out all over the floor. I'm afraid to go down there, it's such a big job. Once the house is straightened and I've gotten things fixed, then we'll go. What's the hurry? I'm going to live a long time!" (He was to be eighty-three that year.)

We knew better. We knew that he wouldn't finish all these things. If they overwhelmed him up to this point, what would change? Instead, we chartered a flight on a private plane for him.

He had never been in a plane before and we thought it was about time. He was always open to new experiences, and this would certainly be an experience he would enjoy. David's brother, John, a pilot, took us up and flew over Mardig's house and other recognizable landmarks-the three domes (horticultural gardens), Brewer's Stadium, and St. Josaphat Basilica. My father enjoyed the whole trip and returned feeling very special because we "went through all this trouble" for him.

Regarding the Eastern European tour, we knew if we were optimistic and kept trying to convince Mardig he would enjoy it, there might be a chance he'd take the trip. Over the long months, it was not to be. His excuses flowed more frequently.

~:   ~

I BEGAN TO THINK A LOT ABOUT HOW WE LIVE CONDITIONAL LIVES. We establish conditions upon ourselves and relationships with others. "*If* you do this, *then* I will...." We also set conditions for doing things *for* ourselves, such as dining at a fine restaurant, traveling to a special place, spending time doing what we truly want to do, etc. "*If* I make a million dollars, *then* I will make time for...."

I have learned that none of us has a guaranteed future. If we need to do something, we should do it now. Other things can wait—the tools in the basement, the house being fixed, the piles of paper, and yes, even taxes! As it was, we had to take care of Mardig's 1993 taxes in 1997!

⌁   ~

DAVID AND I TRIED TO CHANGE OUR APPROACH. We invited Mardig to visit us in California. For three years we tried persuading him to visit. Once a month we'd call and help him visualize how much fun he would have. I own a Miata convertible and had this vision of *cruisin'* the California highways with my father.

I told my sister how much I wished I could buy Mardig new clothes. I could certainly *buy* them, but he wouldn't *wear* them! His clothes were at least twenty years old, and many were forty years old! I just knew how *cool* he'd look in a pair of Dockers pants and a nice crisp cotton print shirt. *Yup, I'd dress 'im like a preppie!* He'd stay with us and father and daughter could bond after so many years of being apart.

⌁   ~

THINGS CHANGED AFTER MY MOTHER DIED. We visited my father and noticed he was no longer taking care of himself. He ignored his cleanliness and nutrition. (My brother still lived with him, but seemed indifferent to Mardig's condition.)

Throughout his life, Mardig didn't care for nutritious food. If someone prepared it, he would eat it; but he never went to a lot of trouble preparing food for himself. He preferred easy-to-make foods. If you went all out and prepared him a gourmet gastronomic delight, you would be disappointed with his review. A hot dog on a bun or a bologna sandwich was just fine.

In contrast, Mardig had always cared about his grooming, at least he did during his working years. Thanks to my mother, his clothes were always clean and neatly pressed. He showered daily, sometimes twice! He always managed a *very* close shave. Nary a stubble appeared due to his attention to detail. And he brushed his teeth for the longest time…much longer than the dental hygienist's recommendation of two minutes.

~   ~

Months passed, and we were aware that Mardig was becoming increasingly disoriented. David, who was on assignment in Wisconsin, took time to care for my father. He sent me the following e-mail in October 1995.

Dear Brenda,

I am at work and I am thinking about your father. I really think that he will soon be near the point where he will no longer be able to take care of himself. I don't think that your sister or brother realize this. Mardig doesn't talk much to them, and they really don't deal much with his day-to-day existence.

The more I think about it, I am sure your father lost about $600 this week, or it could have easily been stolen without him realizing it. It worries me somewhat that with winter coming, he may start a fire in the basement using the incinerator. He is already stockpiling wood down in the basement. I really don't know why.

He really needs someone to spend time with him more and more. I know if something terrible happens to him as a result of his own actions, your brother and sister will wonder how he could have done something so stupid. I guess they don't really talk to him long enough or have the patience to just listen to him speak. If they'd just let him think aloud without leading the conversation, they would see that he is impaired.

I don't know what to do about this situation. I feel that I am in the middle. If I do something to try and help your father, your sister and brother will view it in a negative light because they truly see nothing wrong with him. They don't have the patience or the time to have a normal conversation with him. It is not just his hearing, it's his brain too.

I really feel he needs looking after, and I can only do so much. I was thinking of him all Saturday, Sunday, and today. It is a lot more serious than your brother and sister realize. He may end up killing himself or someone else. He really shouldn't drive anymore.

Sometimes he gets really confused and, one day, he may forget where he lives.

Sorry about this, I just needed to vent.

Love, David

MY FATHER BEGAN HALLUCINATING. He saw my mother. He spoke of my brother bringing a companion into the house. Mardig didn't know this person's name, only that he *looked* like my brother and he helped him carry things out of the house and spent the night when my brother was away on business. He hallucinated these images vividly.

During one of our visits to his home, Mardig told David and me that a little girl and her friends were in the sunroom where he was sitting. We asked where they were now. He said he didn't know. He guessed they went to another part of the house when they heard the doorbell ring. (The little girl really existed. She lived with her mother across the alley behind my father's house.) Mardig shared the details with such clarity that David and I walked through the entire house (basement, first and second floors, and then the attic) before we were convinced that no one else was around.

As his disorientation continued, Mardig stopped doing a lot of things most people take for granted. He stopped taking showers and washing his clothes. On one visit in March 1996, I couldn't bear the smell any longer. I tried very hard to convince him to wash his clothes. He responded with a question, "Why, when I'm working around the house and I'm just going to get dirty?" His reply, when I asked him to shower, "It's cold out. I don't want to take a shower and freeze!" This was his special brand of humor when he felt awkward about something. Instead of saying, "No," he would say something funny.

Chapter 2

CHOICES

1 DECIDED TO VISIT MY FATHER FOR TWO WEEKS DURING THE SUMMER of 1997. Summer is the only time of year I enjoy Milwaukee, because it's not too cold then. I called Mardig and asked if I could visit. Although he did not travel or leave the house much, I did not want to take his availability for granted.

In May, I suggested coming in July. He discouraged me, telling me not to waste my time with him, an old man. He urged me to do my own business and be successful. In this way, he said I would make him proud. He didn't want me to bother with him because that would be a waste of my time. *This was a common view among people of his generation. The children must do their own work and be successful. Never mind the parents. The children's future is what's important.*

He was right in a way. I was working on a consulting contract that would extend into July.

I called in June and suggested I visit in August, to celebrate our birthdays. We were both born on the 22nd of August. After working out the details, I would spend two weeks with him during late August through early September.

❦   ❧

BEFORE I FLEW BACK TO VISIT MARDIG, David and I had lengthy discussions about what we could do for Mardig. We considered many options. We talked with David's parents. We had discussions with our close friends, Sally and Ken, who were taking care of Sally's father (in his early eighties and living in their home); Lew, who was about to retire and move to Mississippi with his wife, Jo, to enjoy the thirty-acre estate they had just purchased; and Dave, who had earned world-wide recognition for being the first person to fly the prototype of the F-22 Raptor, and his wife, Jan, a native Wisconsinite. David's parents and our friends knew us best.

I was about to return to Wisconsin. A decision had to be made. *What were we going to do for Mardig?*

↲ ↳

IN THE BEGINNING, WE SERIOUSLY CONSIDERED HAVING SALLY CARE for my father. She was very kind and helpful to her own father, Pete, in his final years. Although the burden was great, she and Ken managed to provide Pete a nice place to live. Sally has a lot of compassion for the elderly. We addressed the specifics—Sally quitting her job to take this on, payment, what ifs—e.g., what if she quit her established job with full benefits to take care of Mardig and he died in two months? What would happen to her income requirements? What if she and Ken wanted to travel? Mardig would require a lot of attention and care. *We were to learn all too soon to what extent!*

We decided that this was not a reasonable option given Sally's and Ken's plans.

↲ ↳

AFTER TALKING WITH FAMILY, FRIENDS, AND THEN WITH SOCIAL SERVICE workers, city health workers, and nursing home administrators, we had four options.

1. Do nothing. Return to Milwaukee and enjoy the time spent with Mardig knowing that in all likelihood this would be the last time we saw him alive. Milwaukee winters can be harsh. If Mardig became disoriented, he would surely get lost one winter day and literally freeze to death. So the option would be to spend quality time with him, create memories, and then turn my

back on him. *Let my brother and sister worry about him. My brother LIVES WITH HIM! My sister lives five blocks away from him. Why should I be concerned when I live more than 1,800 miles away? Besides, I'm the youngest child and the first one who permanently left home!*

2.   Convince Mardig to move into a nursing facility near his home. This would keep him in a familiar city. Or, move him to a nursing facility in California. Years ago, my mother and father visited California frequently with the dream of living here.

3.   Persuade Mardig to live with us. *All of us agreed this was definitely not a reasonable option!* David and I have no children. We lead very active lives and are involved in many professional pursuits. Our thoughts about starting a family are old-fashioned. One of us must stay home to raise our children because we can't imagine having our children raised by someone else. In the nineteen years we've been together, no children have arrived to alter the course of our lives.

4.   Let Mardig become a ward of the state. When he does something to cause serious danger to himself or others—e.g., leaving an old space heater on and causing a fire, he'd be evaluated and then placed in a county facility. *What a tragedy. I mean, we even rescued three stray cats and brought them into our home! This man is MY FATHER!*

We decided on three options in priority order. First, we'll see if he'll agree to move into a nursing home. If this option doesn't work, we'll just spend memorable time with him and then go home. Finally, as his health deteriorates, the state will step in. We were operating under the assumption that my sister and brother had little interest in him or his affairs. They did not return our calls nor did we receive any support or offer of help when we did talk with them.

Chapter 3

MY LAST VISIT?

This and the next chapter provide a detailed description of how David and I made our decision—one of the most difficult decisions we ever made. Once we decided, we had to quickly carry out our plan. Up until this time, we were unaware that two people could experience so many emotions, so intensely, in such a brief period of time. We didn't sleep. Tossing and turning during the early morning pre-dawn hours, we evaluated the "rightness" of our decision.

In less than fourteen days our lives would dramatically change. We were told that what we accomplished in two weeks usually took several months to a year! We didn't know if this was meant to make us feel better or if it was really true. It did give us some confidence in carrying out our plan.

IN AUGUST, WHEN I SAW MY FATHER AGAIN, he still had not showered or changed his clothes. It was difficult for me to be with him because his smell was quite displeasing. *What was I to do?*

　　　　ᴗ　　　ᴗ

DURING PRIOR MONTHS, WHEN I TALKED WITH MARDIG, in addition to his hallucinations and insistence that he not be a problem for me, *(He is such a humble man.)* he talked about being bothered by "the gas and electric people" who he claimed "were after him." I learned later that he hadn't been paying his bills. Over time, we discovered he let his house insurance lapse.

Mardig was also disoriented about time. The past, present, and future seemed to coexist simultaneously. His mother was living and he was a child living with her. I was a preschool child for whom he was concerned. He would cover a span of forty years at one time!

I had frequent long-distance telephone conversations with the Department of Aging, Milwaukee Social Services, and healthcare workers. I needed a lot of advice. I did not know anything. *Who knows what to do in a situation like this?*

"How do I respond when Mardig hallucinates?"

"Kindly explain to him what is real. Be patient. Be supportive," they advised.

"What might I expect from him?" I shared my thoughts and asked them for ideas regarding my father's care. As the weeks drew closer to my Milwaukee arrival, I set an appointment to visit these agencies to discuss our four options. *They were to give me the one piece of advice that would change my life!*

~: ~

KNOWING I WAS GOING TO RETURN TO MILWAUKEE burdened with these options, Sally loaned me a book entitled, *How Did I Become My Parents' Parent?* by Harriet Sarnoff Schiff. I devoured it voraciously. I needed all the information I could get. I would be in Milwaukee for only two weeks. If I could manage to place Mardig in a nursing home within this time, he would have a chance of survival.

I called my sister and discussed the four options. Surprisingly, she said she'd support my decision. I asked if she would be willing to help. She asked, "How so?" I suggested she could help convince Mardig to move into an assisted-care facility. We then discussed the issues of Mardig safely living at home versus the stress of moving him out of the home he'd occupied for nearly a half-century. I was hopeful that even though my brother showed no interest, at least my sister might get involved.

I called Mardig, and my brother answered the phone. I told him about the option of placing Mardig in an assisted-care facility. His reply, "Mardig doesn't want to go into a nursing home!" Mardig was in the kitchen with him when I called, and I could hear my brother exclaiming to him, "Hey, Mardig! Brenda wants to put you in a nursing home. You wanna go?" This was my brother's special brand of humor.

◡∿   ∿◡

THE DAY DREW NEAR. David and I celebrated my birthday. We also called Mardig and attempted to sing a harmonious rendition of "Happy Birthday" to him.

The following day, August 23, I was awakened by a phone call at 5:39 a.m. *When you have a member of your family who is not well you make a practice of answering the phone since you never know when "the call" will come.*

"We have to talk!" the urgent voice said as it cut into my sleep. "Are you awake?"

"Uh-yeah...yes...yeah. I'm awake," I replied unconvincingly. I tried to make sense of what I was hearing. I had stayed up into the wee hours of the morning brainstorming strategic direction with our business partners. Given the exciting prospects for our future, I had a difficult time getting to sleep. I must have stayed up and worked until 1:45 a.m., just four hours before the call.

"Mardig's been around all night since 1:00 a.m.," the voice continued. "He came here at 7:00 a.m. I told him to go home. I don't want him here! Two days ago, the police picked him up." It was my sister, speaking loudly and commanding my attention.

I was trying to wake up and wondered if something happened to Mardig. Why was she calling me at this inappropriate hour?

She sounded angry, and I was tired. Every time something went wrong, she explained, people called *her*—the authorities, Mardig, social service workers. Every time she tried to contact my brother, he rebuffed her. "I-want-to-see-him-in-a-home!" She shouted each word distinctly.

I couldn't take it any longer. *Each time I suggested we work together, she said she was too busy. Now, she was calling me because she had a problem. Well, I was tired!* I asked her why she was calling me.

Just then I heard her husband telling her that Mardig was at their door again. My sister had reached the end of her rope. She shouted, "I don't want him in this house! Tell him to go home!"

In all fairness, my sister was placed in a bit of a no-win situation. She asked Mardig for keys to his house so she could more easily help him—e.g., get in the house if he needed emergency help. He would not give the keys to her. When he lost his keys or locked himself out, he would come to her. She would help him get into the house (breaking a window) if my brother was unavailable or out of town.

Reasoning that if I offered to help my sister with her perceived problem, she might be more willing to work with me, I asked her how I could help. She said she didn't want anything to do with Mardig. She didn't care if he died. She was sick of taking care of his problems. She had problems of her own. She helped take care of our mother and got nothing. *My brother, who also helped, managed to get a large amount of money transferred to his account. My sister felt shortchanged and not appreciated or rewarded for her efforts.*

After the phone call ended, I sat up awake, aghast. "Why? Why does it have to be like this?" I wondered.

∾   ∾

A FEW DAYS LATER, AFTER I ARRIVED IN MILWAUKEE, my calls and e-mails to my sister went mostly unanswered. I wanted her to attend the meeting I had scheduled with the Department of Aging representative. When she did answer, she was "much too busy" to get together with me.

I realized I was on my own. I was not going to get the help I needed from my sister or brother. I also realized later that this may be a good thing—*I wouldn't get any interference.*

∾   ∾

I ARRANGED TO STAY WITH JOHN, DAVID'S BROTHER, his wife, Anna, and Finn, their Springer Spaniel.

After I arrived in Milwaukee I went to my father's house. His house was uncomfortably warm and smelled musty. The drapes were drawn and we had to turn on the lights to see. I suggested we sit outside. We decided to sit on the cement steps in the back of the house. Mardig went to the garage to get some foam padding to place on the steps for us to sit on.

I looked around. The house was the same—neglected, worn, and tired. It was sad to see that the grandeur of what was once a bank president's home was long gone. My father was the second owner. The yard was in desperate need of attention. One could only guess what flora and fauna were inhabiting this overgrown urban ecosystem!

Yet, I enjoyed sitting outside on the back steps. Years ago, while my mother watered her vegetable garden, I sat on the same steps smelling the freshly watered plants. Sometimes if the wind blew just right, I would be tickled by a light cool mist.

I looked around. The garden had long been unattended. It was now a lush array of weeds with the exception of four trees—my father's famous apple tree, my mother's pear tree, and the two evergreen seedlings my mother planted shortly before her death. They were about a foot tall when she planted them. As I looked at them now, they stood over eight feet tall.

Mardig and I sat on the steps and talked about anything that came to mind. We started with family members' names, how they were related, and who was still living. I got confused when he spoke of his wife and mother. He would refer to both as "Ma" as if they were the same person. I found it difficult to keep track of whether he was speaking about his mother or my mother.

Since his Meals on Wheels lunch was to arrive before 1:00 p.m., he asked that we continue our conversation on the front steps of the house. He didn't want to miss his lunch. The Social Services or Health Department had arranged for this service after they had visited Mardig a few times and saw his sparsely filled refrigerator and observed that he wasn't eating properly.

When his meal arrived, we went inside so he could eat. Since there was no other food in the house, he urged me to share his food. I felt strange partaking of his small meal—nourishment he depended upon. I could easily get in my car and pick up some food. It was more difficult for him.

Still, I opted to accept his invitation and we shared his meal over more conversation.

I looked inside his refrigerator. All I saw was a gallon of milk and two half-gallons of orange juice. One had a label with my brother's name on it. The other container was on the bottom shelf. This must have been Mardig's juice. When I picked it up I noticed it had expired. I pulled out the container, drained the contents into the sink, much to my father's objections, and threw the empty bottle into the trash.

I became concerned that Mardig would get sick from eating spoiled food. I told him I wanted to go grocery shopping because there was nothing to eat in the house. He agreed and said he would accompany me, adding that he wanted me to be comfortable. *He wanted* me *to be comfortable and have food. I wanted* him *to have food!* He told me he had to get his wallet because he wanted to pay. I told him it was not necessary. He insisted, explaining that I was his guest and he wanted to take care of me. So I waited for him to find his wallet. When he did, we went to the store. At the store he realized he only had $11. I picked up the tab and accepted his $10. He wanted to save one dollar in case of an emergency.

We returned with a variety of easy-to-prepare foods—bologna, fresh bread, chocolate pudding, an assortment of chewy cookies, fresh milk and juice, bananas, grapes, tomatoes, soda, and beer (for me). His refrigerator was now better stocked. Even I could nibble on a few things.

⌁   ∾

MARDIG ASKED TO VISIT MY SISTER. He wanted to see us together. I suggested that we call her instead. *Experience told me that if we knocked on her door, she would not open it. Never mind that she hadn't returned my calls, letters, or e-mails. Never mind that I traveled so many miles to visit.* He asked that I call her. I said, "No." I wasn't ready to be rejected just yet. Besides, I wanted to enjoy the visit with my father a little longer.

So he called her. He couldn't hear too well. As her answering machine played her telephone greeting (she screened her calls) he thought it was actually her and he began to speak. He became confused when the voice kept talking and then he heard a long beep. He managed to leave a message.

We then went into his room, where he liked to work at his desk.

The phone rang. I suggested that he get it. I listened to see if it was for me. I had given his number to the Health Department and the Department of Aging representatives and my friends.

I could hear the voice. It was my sister. I thought I would talk with her if she sounded in a good mood.

"Mardig, are you all right?" she asked.

"Yes."

"Wha'cha doin'?" she asked playfully.

"I have company."

"Who?"

I urged Mardig not to divulge his secret, that his company was me.

"Come by and see."

"Mardig, who?" she inquired in a concerned voice.

"Come by and see!" he toyed, holding his ground.

"Mardig, I have things to do!" she replied, in an irritated manner.

"C'mon just for a few minutes," he pleaded. (She lived only five blocks away.)

"Mardig, I have to take [her husband] to work."

This went nowhere. I was glad I hadn't spoken with her. I had heard these excuses too many times before. Even while I write this, my anxiety increases and I feel my muscles tighten. Excuses, excuses, excuses—while life passes us by!

⌁   ∾

MARDIG AND I RESUMED OUR DISCUSSION. I urged him to let me look into alternatives for his care. I suggested he consider living in a place where people could help him. I recommended he consider having someone live with him. I told him I was concerned for him, that it was getting harder for him to manage everything by himself. I reminded him that he had gotten lost and that the police had to bring him home. I added that the Department of Health and Human Services and the Department of Aging had case files on him and were moni-toring his care.

He laughed and asked, "Me? Why would all these people be con-cerned about me?"

I explained he was a risk to himself because he got disoriented. I told him that some day kids who wanted to make trouble might see him walking on the street and hurt him. Hesitatingly, I added that he may not survive the winter. He could freeze to death.

We then spoke of dying. Mardig shared his perspective.

"Millions of people die each year. We're like animals...we keep crawling until we stop."

I disagreed with him. I explained that I could not accept his per-spective because he was my father.

"After I die it doesn't matter," he said.

I couldn't argue with this. He had a point.

～   ～

WHAT WAS I TO DO? If we pulled him out of his house he might die because he had nothing to live for. At least everything was familiar in his home. He could tinker with his tools and work on things he'd been working on for a long time. People live long lives because they per-ceive they have a purpose, they believe they have something to do. Take this away from them and their reason for living goes away too. Could I accept the risk of removing Mardig from the place he had called home for so long—so he that he would have a chance of living through the winter? What if the move was too much for him to bear and he died a few months later? Would I be able to face myself then?

This was not about *me*, I reminded myself. This was not about what would be *convenient* for *me*. This had to be what was *best* for *him*, what would work for him.

The following day I was to meet with the Department of Aging representative. I eagerly looked forward to this meeting because I needed answers. I prepared for the meeting with one-and-a-half pages of questions evenly spaced on graph paper. I was excited at the prospect that in less than twenty-four hours my questions would be answered. I envisioned leaving the meeting with a clear sense of direction.

The outcome of this meeting would change our lives.

⌐   ⌐

I CALLED MY SISTER THE EVENING BEFORE MY MEETING with the Department of Aging. I left the following message on her answering machine: "On Friday when we talked, you said you'd return my calls. I'm now in Milwaukee. Please call me at…." I received no return call that night or the next day. I had hoped she could join me at the Department of Aging.

I met with the Department of Aging representative alone. Given the options I faced and our family situation, the representative suggested I encourage my father to move into an assisted-care facility. Since I had spent the day before trying to persuade Mardig of the benefits of moving into an assisted-care facility, without much success, I doubted I would be successful in convincing him of this option. Still, the representative might have greater insight than I did. I asked her how I could persuade him. She recommended I approach my father with the benefits of moving into such a facility—for example, twenty-four-hour staff to take care of his needs, and friends with whom to socialize. I inquired as to the possibility of causing trauma by moving Mardig out of familiar surroundings. She agreed that trauma to my father was a potential risk. I asked for additional options.

She encouraged me to find assisted care for my father, since he could still manage himself and his own affairs. She thought a companion to live with him would be a good idea. David and I considered this too, but we heard stories of live-in caregivers taking advantage of the elderly. So this would be a last resort. I asked for other options.

She suggested going to court to get a conservatorship. I asked what this was. She explained that a person deemed incompetent can have a court-appointed conservator to handle his/her affairs. This places responsibility and accountability of the individual on the conservator. I did not think Mardig was incompetent. *At least, I wasn't ready to admit it. I wanted to preserve as much of his independence and dignity as he deserved.* Just to be sure though, I asked if she thought he was incompetent. "No," she replied, "he was 'on the fence,' but as the disease progressed, he would eventually be unable to take care of himself or make decisions."

"Could I be a court-appointed conservator even though I lived in California?" I asked.

She said, "No." Either my sister or brother would have to be Mardig's conservator. My sister and brother were not options. They hadn't helped Mardig so far—and I doubted this would change.

"What other options are there?" I asked.

She said another option was to ask my father to appoint me his attorney. *What did this mean?*

She suggested I get a power of attorney for his affairs and his healthcare.

I told her my father had granted me power of attorney over his bank accounts. "Wasn't this enough?" I asked.

"No," she said. "You'll need one to manage all his affairs and healthcare."

What was she talking about? Do I have to represent my father in court?

She explained that a power of attorney (POA) gives an individual the right to take care of the grantor's affairs within the limits expressed in the document.

My heart sank. On one hand I felt a childlike excitement of being appointed a high level of responsibility—an "attorney" no less! After all, I was the baby of the family. The youngest family member never got any respect! Wow, I was about to do a very grown-up thing. It was like getting behind the wheel of a car for the first time. It was like buying my first house. I felt grown-up. On the other hand, I felt a dreadful sinking feeling. I should have listened to this feeling.

I really wished my sister and brother would get involved. Since I wasn't having any luck contacting them or getting them involved, maybe the Department of Aging representative could help. Since she thought it would be best if my brother, sister, and I went to Mardig and encouraged him to let us help him, she volunteered to call my brother and sister to encourage them to follow up with me. She added that all of us could get a POA for Mardig.

I thought this would be a good idea. This way, *all* of us would be involved. Later I learned from other caregivers, it would *not* be a good idea to have *all* of us share a power of attorney. The responsibilities of a shared POA required a lot of coordinating and agreement. *I couldn't even get my brother and sister to return my calls. I was told they didn't return the Department of Aging representative's calls either.*

⌐   ∾

THE FOLLOWING DAY I CALLED MY SISTER AGAIN. *I couldn't give up. I was hopeful!* She answered the phone. Her voice caught me off guard, since she usually let the answering machine take her calls. I asked her to help coordinate Mardig's affairs while I was in Milwaukee. She told me all the things she had to do. She said that the building inspector was on her back. *I'd heard this excuse for three and a half years, even while my mother was alive! Milwaukee either had a very patient building inspector or my sister had a very strong back!* I urged her to get involved. I reminded her of the times she said she received the brunt of the requests and asked for my help, even though I was in California. I suggested that she use me while I was in Milwaukee. She continued giving me excuses. My frustration with these excuses increased. For years I had witnessed her concern with herself. With these thoughts rushing past me, as she told me how busy she was, I became impatient. I told her I observed she couldn't make any commitments. After a moment longer, of what I perceived to be annoying excuses, I hung up the telephone. *I hate doing this. It's such an immature thing to do, to just put the phone down without acknowledging the conclusion of a conversation.*

⌐   ∾

ADVICE! I NEED ADVICE! I e-mailed Sally. She suggested I hire an attorney to send my sister a letter inviting her to be involved. This way, the letter would be on record, as would her lack of involvement. This was a precaution since I did not know what to expect of my family.

My sister had informed me earlier that my brother was considering having Mardig committed. I didn't like the sound of this, especially since Mardig and my brother did not get along very well. My experience had been that my sister and brother were nowhere to be found when there was work to be done. Yet, when the work was finished, they were quick to judge the outcome. So, it was better to be safe than sorry. *How do I find an attorney?*

I called the Department of Aging representative and left a message requesting her help in finding an attorney. I also asked David to fly back over Labor Day weekend to help me. I was getting nowhere, and I wanted to accomplish something during this visit. David might be able to talk some sense into Mardig. After all, my father respected David because he was a *man*!

David flew into Milwaukee. After meeting him at the airport we visited my father. The next few days can best be described as a whirlwind.

Mardig enjoyed visiting with David. They talked up a storm. In fact, my father was unaware that David had ever left town! Meanwhile, I went down to the basement. I'd been debating whether the unusual smell from the basement was mildew or something more serious. I later mentioned the smell to David, and we checked it out together. He didn't smell anything unusual. "I think it's gas," I said. *Women have a keener sense of smell than men.* Since I had noticed a gas leak at our home, David encouraged me to call the gas company.

The gas company representative said he'd have someone come immediately. When the representative arrived, he located major gas leaks. This was alarming because, when we thought about it, we realized we had smelled the same odor during our visit in March. Could it have been leaking this long?

It was a good thing Mardig didn't smoke. A flame could have blown the whole place to smithereens! And Mardig had been delinquent paying his house insurance! By the time everything was done, it took five workers one day to tear up the front brickwork to get at the leaking valve and to seal the gas lines in the house. *Wasn't my brother living in this house?*

David and I decided we had a mission to care for Mardig. The gas leak and the empty refrigerator were illustrative of his neglect. We couldn't turn our backs on him. We had to do something for him. We began with the simple things—cleaning him up. The following evening, when Mardig grew weary and removed his clothes to go to bed, I grabbed the clothes he had not washed since March and washed them.

We also tried to contact my brother. He had not returned earlier calls or faxes to his office. We had no other way of contacting him since he still hadn't shown up at home.

While clearing some piles of papers, we found a magazine with a woman's name on it. We heard that my brother had a girlfriend, so we went with this lead. We found an address in another suburb and decided to visit the following day to track down my brother. Our search was fruitless.

That evening, while going through more of Mardig's papers, we found some U.S. Savings Bonds stashed in a business envelope discreetly hidden between a couple of books. The three rubber bands which had once tightly bound the bonds were now dried out and stuck to the bonds. We peeled off the rubber bands and then alerted Mardig of the bonds. He said to put them aside and he'd look at them later. David, who had spent a year-and-a-half with my father, knew what this meant. He would place them somewhere and then they'd get lost again. *Everything would be looked at later...decided later.* So, we took them. This too was a risk. What if we lost them? We did not take this responsibility lightly and we were nervous about what we had done.

We had taken the first serious step in becoming actively involved in my father's life.

Chapter 4

OUR LIVES ARE ABOUT TO CHANGE

*D*AVID AND I SPENT THE NEXT FEW DAYS SORTING THROUGH Mardig's papers. We began to get a better picture of the seriousness of the situation. Meanwhile, Mardig was enjoying our genuine interest and began to reflect on his past. I had never learned much about his past. I knew more about my mother's side of the family. Mardig did not share a lot about his family. Old misunderstandings had kept the families apart. So this discovery process became an archeological dig. I was on an expedition to learn about an important part of my family history.

Since David would only be in Milwaukee during the weekend, our time was limited. Nonetheless, we did take a few hours off to enjoy something that made Milwaukee famous—beer! Sprecher Brewery, a micro-brewery in Milwaukee, was sponsoring their annual Sprecherfest, their version of an Oktoberfest. We went with David's brother, John, and his wife, Anna. We sampled nearly all of the beers, and then ordered more of the two brews we liked best. As the evening hours passed and we enjoyed *many* glasses of beer, we found ourselves getting philosophical about my father.

Alcohol does unexpected things to people. Sprecherfest and great beer! *We decided to have my father live with us!*

Ahhh, alcohol...its inhibition-reducing effects have surprised many couples who, months later, learn they are about to become parents. We too decided to become parents. We decided to adopt an eighty-six year old man—my father.

⌐   ⌐

WE HAD TO CONVINCE MARDIG OF OUR INTENTIONS. This was the hard part. We took it slowly. We asked him a lot of "what if" questions. "What if you were to move to California?"

He didn't think it was a good idea because he thought he needed money. "Where would I live?" he asked.

"You would stay with us," we said.

He didn't seem to be really excited about that. He was very independent and wanted to be sure he could take care of himself. We reminded him of the bonds we had found, some $28,000 in face value. *We had no idea what these thirty-year-old bonds would be worth.* We also reminded Mardig he had some General Electric stock; although we did not know how much. And we knew he had a few certificates of deposit. We estimated he was worth a couple hundred thousand, and we told him this. He laughed.

⌐   ⌐

THE WEEKEND WAS SOON OVER AND DAVID HAD TO RETURN TO California. I stayed and found more of Mardig's essential paperwork. Each time I found something official-looking regarding his finances, I shared it with him. These included bank statements, dividend earnings statements, and savings bonds. He began to get an idea of what he owned, and then he began to have hope. He was surprised he could have amassed this much. *So was I! We were raised very frugally.*

I made a deal with Mardig. I told him if he really had this much money, he would have to come out to California and stay with us. Now this may sound strange. But his fiercely independent nature made him constantly question what would become of him if he didn't have enough money. My assurances did not allay his deep-rooted concern and need for independence and self-sufficiency. So I was relieved when he finally accepted my offer. I excitedly e-mailed a note to David and to Sally and Ken.

Sally replied first. Considering the options we had discussed earlier, we really caught her off guard with our final decision. Here's an excerpt from her e-mail to me:

> WOW!!!!!!! This turn I did not expect.
> OK: Are you sure you can handle this? You will be questioning every move you make from now on. You are your father's parent. You have a lot to do.…I am in total shock, I just didn't expect this. Just wanted you to know I read your message and Ken and I will be here for you and David. Lord have mercy…If you need the van to pick up you and your dad at the airport just let us know…I believe in you, you'll do just fine.
> Love, Sally

Usually when I returned to Milwaukee, I visited my friends. On this trip, I had also planned to accomplish a little business. Everything changed. I did not have time to visit my friends or conduct my business. I still had not been able to contact my brother. My sister and I were no longer communicating. I was on my own. I had to take care of all the affairs by myself and get Mardig ready to move to California. *What do you take on the plane? He has a lot of things he likes—his tools, familiar clothes, grooming supplies, and paperwork. Where do I begin? What's enough? What will happen to the house?*

I was becoming overwhelmed by the responsibilities. There were a lot of loose ends to be tied…one of them was Mardig's vacillations on whether he'd accompany me to California or not. *Oh, and I still had to buy the plane ticket.* I had to follow up on the POA. Who would I call? I didn't know any attorneys who did this type of work. I had called the Department of Aging representative on Friday and left a message. She called after the Labor Day weekend and said that the Department had a prepared a list of attorneys who specialized in elder law and she would be happy to give me the list. I went to her office that afternoon and picked up the list. The following day, I made a few phone calls. By the time I found an attorney who would be able to help me it was Thursday. Only four days remained before my two weeks were up and I had to return home.

⌐   ～

I WAS CONCERNED ABOUT WHAT I WAS DOING—taking my father to California. I couldn't help but feel I might be doing something wrong. *It is the wretched fear of all the youngest children in families. I was no different. Even though my brother, sister, and I were not communicating, this was also their father I was relocating.*

I needed to make sure Mardig would authorize my efforts to help him in some legal fashion. I was uncertain of my brother's and sister's reactions and didn't want them to accuse me of anything. If I was going to take care of my father's affairs, I needed to do it *right*.

Up until now, Mardig still had not showered. He could not go out in public this way. He was dirty, and he smelled. I guessed that he had not taken a shower since March, when I last saw him. How was I going to get him to take a shower?

I used the best line of reasoning I could. Since Mardig was appreciative of having me around to help him, I explained that if he wanted me to take care of his affairs we would have to do it legally, which meant seeing an attorney. I added that I would not feel comfortable about him meeting an attorney when he smelled so bad. He asked me if he really did smell bad. I said, "Yes." *I liked talking candidly with my father. He was a rational man and did not seem to be offended when he knew my comments were for his own good.*

He surprised me and said, "For you, I will. Now, we need to get me some clean clothes." I assured him that if he would start his shower, I would gather his clothes and have them ready for him. He said "Okay," and went upstairs to take his shower. Just then, the phone rang. It was the attorney with some last minute questions about the POA. He wanted to draft the document so we could review it when we arrived at his office. Just as I hung up the phone, Mardig walked into the living room wearing only a loosely buttoned shirt, no pants, no underwear. I averted my glance and asked, "Why aren't you upstairs taking your shower?"

He said, "Because you said you'd bring me some clean clothes."

I said, "I will. Please go up and take your shower."

I felt strange seeing my father this way. I had never seen him naked (even partially) before. I urged him to go upstairs again. He walked toward me and stood in front of me. He said he felt very close to me and that he knew I was trying to take care of him, and that he loved me.

I began feeling uncomfortable. If he were fully dressed, I could accept this. But with only a shirt on, which did a poor job of covering his private parts, I did not know how to interpret this. As awkward as I felt, I took his hand, being careful not to look at him, and asked him to come upstairs with me. I reminded him that I wanted him to take a shower. He asked me to help him. I hesitated, and then a voice inside of me said, "If you want him to shower, just help him. It took you six months to get him to this point!" I turned on the water as he undressed. I tried hard to focus only on the water and the faucet. Once the water was warm, I assisted him into the shower taking great care to avert my eyes away from his nakedness. I closed the shower curtain and told him I would be leaving the bathroom. *Phew! That was weird! I had never had such an experience.*

I went downstairs to find some clothes. He had a lot of nice clothes he no longer wore. I quietly entered the bathroom, while he was still showering, and placed his clothes inside. After he finished his shower, he called my name. I hesitantly stood by the bathroom door. "Yes?" I asked.

"How do I look?" he asked.

I didn't know what to expect. I slowly opened the door and saw Mardig sitting in his undershirt and boxers on the toilet. He was putting on his socks. I looked at him. Wow, he looked so clean and fresh. I was proud of him. *Still, what had just happened lingered in my mind.*

～   ～

ON THE WAY TO THE ATTORNEY'S OFFICE, which was only a mile away, I began feeling afraid. I was scared of the unknown. I didn't know what to expect. This was such a grown-up thing to do. I was with my father, about to sign legal documents to handle his affairs. He had been so very private about his affairs. I knew nothing except for the details he had shared during the past several years.

We arrived at the attorney's office, which was located on the second floor of a neighborhood bank on the south side of Milwaukee. The receptionist greeted us and asked us to have a seat. We barely had enough time to digest the office suite—the solid woodwork and tall ceilings characterized by some of Milwaukee's older buildings, before Attorney Cohn appeared and invited us into his office. He introduced himself, shook our hands, and invited us to sit. Even though Mardig was sitting next to me, I still felt nervous. After all, this was a serious responsibility.

I looked around at the mounds of paperwork, files, and books everywhere. A touch of pity competed with my nervousness as I wondered how this attorney would ever get through all this paperwork. Yet, Attorney Cohn was organized enough to have completed a draft power of attorney document. Only the details had to be reviewed. I had to give him credit for his efficiency. Yet I couldn't shake the uneasiness I felt. This was an entirely new experience and I had no idea what I was getting myself into.

David, as I came to refer to Attorney Cohn, must have sensed my discomfort. He tried to put me at ease with what I would later discover was his special brand of *very dry* humor.

He was in his late forties, wore rimless glasses, and had locks of lightly salt and peppered curly hair. He sported colorful suspenders with bold, colorful neckties. Contrasting these vibrant accessories was his starched pima cotton shirt, which gave him an air of professionalism. It was almost as if one foot was firmly implanted in the 1960s and the other, in the 1990s. His disarming style helped me relax a little, despite my uncertainties.

David turned to Mardig and asked him questions about his (my father's) intentions.

"Do you know why you are here?"

"Yes, to have my daughter manage my affairs."

"Is this your daughter?"

"Yes, this is my daughter." Mardig beamed when he looked at me.

"What's her name?"

"Brenda."

"Can you please review these documents and let me know if you have any questions? I'll explain some of the parts to you."

Mardig didn't want to read all the pages that were put before us and handed the documents to me to look at "Since you are now managing my affairs," he jokingly added.

What if I was doing the wrong thing? My head kept telling me to grow up and get through it. I did not pay attention to what my body was telling me. *Don't do it! It's more trouble than you can possibly imagine! Don't do it! It will turn your life upside down! Don't do it! It will totally change the course of your life!*

I insisted that Mardig look through the power of attorney documents with me. I didn't understand everything. In fact, I'm not certain I read the entire document. I asked a few questions and then David Cohn drew our attention to other important parts of the document. We spent considerable time going over the healthcare power of attorney. Mardig asked me if I thought they were acceptable. Still nervous and feeling mixed emotions, I said, "Yes." I signed them and so did my father. *After all, Attorney Cohn was on the list provided by the Department of Aging. He had to be good.*

David then asked Mardig if he understood what he had just signed.

"Yes, my daughter is my attorney!" he replied looking at me and patting my knee.

～　　～

THIS STEP WAS BEHIND US. We were finished at the attorney's office. What next? My feelings of being overwhelmed began to suffocate me.

We went grocery shopping. Mardig had eaten the food we bought earlier. While I walked up and down the aisles, I noticed a special buoyancy about him. He seemed so childish and playful. I asked him how he felt, and he said he was really happy. He added that he felt I was going to help him and that I really cared for him. This gave me a warm feeling. He said he loved me. I liked hearing him say this, but then there was that shower incident earlier which gave me mixed feelings. He added, "I love you so much, I want to eat you!" He said this really loud. I started getting embarrassed. He said it a few more times, and I asked him to stop, that I was feeling embarrassed. He said, "Okay."

It was like a major weight had been lifted off of him. He had relinquished control. I wasn't sure how I felt about this. On one hand, I felt honored. On the other, I felt a great sense of responsibility…which scared me.

⌐   ⌐

I CALLED SALLY FOR A PERSPECTIVE ON THE SHOWER INCIDENT with my father. She shared her experiences with her incontinent father. After forty-five minutes, I started feeling stronger and able to go on. I still needed to get Mardig's medical records. I had to find his doctor first.

A few days later, I sent Sally the following e-mail of my progress.

> It has been very difficult with my father. I am trying to move much more quickly than he is comfortable. When I return Tuesday, the 10th, I hope to have him with me!
>
> David and I are trying to take this one step at a time. It's like adopting a child. Everything in our lives will change. We can't come and go as freely as we have. And we need to form proper eating habits so my father can have regular and nutritious meals! As it is, David and I lead such a hectic pace, we only eat once a day! We'll even have to get someone to care for him when both David and I are away. Since he'll be in a strange and unfamiliar place, we'd hate to see him wander and get lost! Oh well, one step at a time!

⌐   ⌐

IT WAS THE MORNING OF SEPTEMBER 10, the last day I'd be in Milwaukee, when I sent an e-mail to a business associate to explain why we could not meet. The following is an excerpt:

> …imagine getting a man, who's lived in the same house for 45 years to move to Los Angeles on such short notice. I've had to, in this brief time (one week), find a local attorney, get a power of attorney, locate and speak with my father's doctor, obtain copies of my father's medical records, take care of him day-to-day given

the soon-to-be upheaval of his life…in short, I've managed to get by on 4 - 5 hours of sleep and take care of his affairs the rest of the time.

·∾·   ∾

AT APPROXIMATELY 7:00 P.M. IN MILWAUKEE the sun was setting and my father and I boarded Midwest Express for Los Angeles. This was his first commercial flight. Mardig couldn't fathom the idea that he was flying six to seven miles above the ground. Also, he couldn't imagine such a good meal would be served on a plane. (Midwest Express flies entirely first class and the meals are exquisite.) In fact, he didn't believe he was flying in a plane.

Anyway, he wouldn't believe me when I told him how high we were flying, so he got up to ask the flight attendants. He stood at the front of the plane for a good portion of the flight, talking with them. I think they were so taken by Mardig's innocence and genuine kindness, that they entertained him for nearly an hour. And then they gave him his wings.

David and I had just become parents.

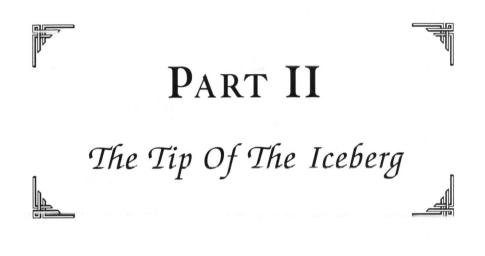

PART II

The Tip Of The Iceberg

When you decide to do something, you have to see it through. Over a few pitchers of beer, we decided to invite my father to live with us. We had to see it through. There was no changing our minds. We could not turn away from the responsibility we now faced. So, we prepared ourselves to care for Mardig. David had taken great care to prepare Mardig's room in our home. He bought things my father would need, such as toiletries, more clothes than the few I had purchased while in Milwaukee, and food for healthy, balanced meals.

Others view David and me as strong planners. The advantage of this is that we are rarely surprised by events because we think through all the details in advance. The disadvantage is that we stay awake nights, churning out the details in our minds, making sure we've covered all the bases with the information we have. Even so, we could not foresee the magnitude of the responsibility we had undertaken.

Caring for my father was only a portion of the responsibilities we faced. There were many tasks we had to follow up on, such as getting a Social Security card for him. (He had lost this and any other forms of identification.) The Social Security representative suggested we get a California ID card for him. We couldn't apply for one without a birth certificate, citizenship papers, or a Social Security card.

We had to follow up on his healthcare. We had to find a local doctor who specialized in Alzheimer's disease.

We tried to open a local bank account for him, and were told we couldn't open one without a California ID or a Social Security card.

We still had mounds of Mardig's paperwork that we had packed and had shipped to California to look through. He had kept so many records, we were unable to process everything at his home in Milwaukee. During subsequent visits to Milwaukee, we gathered important documents and air-freighted them by registered mail to California.

Following up on, making sense of, and organizing all this paperwork proved to be our biggest nightmare. We were shocked at what we found. Our thoughts were so dominated by Mardig's affairs that we often existed in a daze. Once, while driving on a familiar road, I momentarily lost my sense of direction and forgot where I was! Attorney David Cohn summarized it best with the following analogies: "You decided to pick up an acorn and got the whole oak tree! You decided to pick up one grain of sand and got the whole beach!"

Chapter 5

OUR LIVES TAKE AN
UNEXPECTED TURN

O<small>NCE WE LANDED IN LOS ANGELES, MARDIG WAS HAPPY</small> to see David. He and David talked for an hour and a half, all the way home. I closed my eyes and fell asleep in the backseat of the car. I was exhausted.

At 11:00 p.m., after a six-hour trip (four-hour flight and two hours for baggage retrieval and the drive home), my father grew increasingly disoriented and repeatedly insisted that he wanted to go home. He promised that he would visit us the following day, but for now, he'd like to return home for the night. *What were we to do?* We explained how far he had traveled. It took us another hour and a half to persuade him to spend the night. We said we'd take him home in the morning. *What started as a kind gesture on our part might be shortened by Mardig's desire to return home. We decided that if he really wanted to return to Milwaukee, we would fly back with him the following day.*

The next morning, he was well rested. We greeted him with breakfast. After having only one balanced meal every weekday from the Meals on Wheels program, he was delighted to sit down to a hearty breakfast of eggs, bread, cheese, and grapefruit. *So were we! We rarely ate breakfast. But we had to change our routine. We had Mardig to care for now.*

I took him for a drive around the neighborhood. Since we had arrived at night, I wanted him to see as much as possible during the day. I wasn't entirely convinced he understood where he was. He liked the houses and the neighborhood. He had so much energy! Having worked so intensely for the last two weeks in Milwaukee, with very little sleep, all I could think of was getting some rest and catching up on all the work that had accumulated in my absence. Sensing my exhaustion and desire to get some work done, David asked Mardig if he'd like to go for a walk.

"Yes," Mardig said.

Mardig loved to walk and it helped him get familiar with his new surroundings. They put on their shoes and left for what David promised would be at least a forty-five minute walk. *Ahhh. Peace. Quiet. Relaxation.*

I never heard from my sister while I was in Milwaukee, so I called and left a telephone message for her the morning after I returned to California. I felt uncomfortable that she wasn't involved and that she hadn't responded to my calls. Despite my feelings, I sent an e-mail to her. I knew she would at least read a note from me. I tried to sound as upbeat as possible.

> Subject: MARDIG
>
> Hi!
>
> Hey, I left a message on your answering machine this morning…it was shortly before 1:00 p.m. your time.
>
> I managed to persuade Mardig to come to California with me. The logistics were no easy feat! Taking a man on an airplane (his first commercial flight—by the way, he earned his WINGS which the flight attendants pinned on his jacket) and leaving a home he's lived in for 45 years.
>
> I bought him clothes (you know how dirty and worn his clothes were) pants, shirts, PJs, underwear, and socks and got him to take a shower (after five months without one?). Actually, I wish you could have seen him, HE LOOKS PRETTY COOL!
>
> So he's here and I'm one tired puppy! He really needs a lot of looking after…especially since he is in unfamiliar territory. I took him for a drive and then David went with him for a walk.
>
> Well, this is all I will share with you for now. Hope his being out

here provides you a brief respite. By the way, I haven't reached
[our brother] yet…his reaction should be interesting.

Tryin' to do what I can for Mardig,

Brenda

I knew in my heart that David and I were going to take this journey without the support of my sister or brother, so I began updating
my friends and colleagues, soliciting their advice. I communicated
mostly by e-mail. This was helpful because people could read their
messages when it was convenient for them. They wouldn't have to listen to long-winded telephone messages that begged for advice, understanding, pity, compassion, or sympathy. One of my e-mails was to a
colleague who had moved to San Diego. I had promised to visit him
in his new home once I returned from Milwaukee.

Subject: HELLO FROM CALIFORNIA!

Rodger,

Helloooooo…I'm Baaaaack! Uh-ohhhh.

Update: I have brought my father out here to live with David
and me. So, this'll put a little different spin on things—freedom,
accessibility, sleep (he wanders at night)…David and I take turns
getting up and taking twenty minutes or so to talk him into going
back to sleep. Hey, it's like havin' a BABY!

Once things settle a little bit then we'll see how I can work out
a trip to your neck o' the woods (oops, beach!). I'll bring you a
cigar. (It's a BOY!)

I hope you are settling in nicely and that you've been at a beer
race already!

Brenda Avadian

Speaker, Author, & Human Development Consultant

During breakfast, one weekend morning, Mardig shared his appreciation for our care and wanted to know why we were going out of
our way for him. I told him because he is my father and reminded him
of the power of attorney he had granted. He smiled at the idea that we
would care for him *simply* because he was my father. He then asked if
I had the POA papers. I said, "Yes," and went into his room to get
them for him. He read them for about thirty minutes and then spoke.

"The person who wrote this is not *just* an attorney, but *an attor-*

ney!" he emphasized. He then asked, "So I've appointed you to take care of *every*thing?" He emphasized *every*.

"Yes," I hesitatingly replied, uncertain where this was leading.

"Good," he said much to my relief. "Now I don't have to worry about *any*thing!"

I sent an e-mail to David Cohn to update him on how Mardig was doing in California, and to give him my father's feedback on the POA he authored. I also informed him that I still had not heard from my sister or brother, and asked him to follow up on some unfinished business—determining who owned the home Mardig just left. *My brother had repeatedly told my sister that our father's house was his (my brother's). We needed to check this out.*

Later, Mardig brought up the subject of his finances. "Okay, we have an account in Omaha. We need to get that money."

"All right, we'll do that," I replied. Time to get busy. *When will I ever get my own work done?*

～   ～

DURING THE FOLLOWING WEEKS I MADE MANY PHONE CALLS and sent and received a lot of e-mails. The first calls I placed were to my neighbors. Despite the potential embarrassment of letting others know I was caring for my father, whom I may not be able to control, I told them the truth: David and I had adopted my eighty-six-year-old father, who was diagnosed with dementia of the Alzheimer's type. He's about 5'1" and 112 pounds. (He had lost a lot of weight before we became involved in his life.) He typically wears black-rimmed glasses, a baseball cap, and a brown jacket. If you see him on the street please call us because he is not familiar with the area and could get lost easily.

This proved to be helpful. Two days later one of our neighbors called to say she just saw my father walking toward her house.

～   ～

IT IS AMAZING HOW WHEN YOUR LIFE CHANGES it impacts the entire fabric of your relationships with other people. In our case, it not only affected our personal relationships but our professional ones as well.

One colleague wrote to us and said that what David and I were doing was a noble act, and that given her experience with her uncle, it's like having a child. My reply:

> Thank you for your kind words. Yes, he is David's and my 86-year old son. We will give him a safe place to live his life with dignity.
>
> We have learned to go without a full night of sleep…as with a child, we must get up periodically and cajole him back to sleep.
>
> He also gets very confused when he returns after we take him out. I like him to be stimulated, yet I can begin to see why so many elderly are placed into nursing homes and drugged into sedation. If he wasn't my father, I doubt David and I could be so patient with him. As you may suspect, we have slowed down tremendously since he's come into our lives.

I did not know it at the time, but my decision to take care of my father would alter my life significantly. I would not be able to see this colleague until one year later. More importantly, I stopped using my "Speaker, Author, & Consultant" signature block when sending e-mails. Mardig's affairs had so dominated my life I could no longer travel to fulfill my speaking and consulting obligations.

A former colleague wrote:

> David and you are extraordinary folks—not everyone can accept the work and responsibility involved in caring for an Alzheimer's relative, even a beloved member of the family. I tip my hat to you both.

Another colleague and his wife, who are two of the most disciplined people I know, wrote: (excerpted)

> Taking your father under your care will certainly be a challenge, and we commend you for your faith and concern…most people would not want nor be willing to make such a stretch.

They weren't kidding!

Chapter 6

ADULT DAY CARE

*D*URING THIS TIME, WE STARTED THE *REAL* RESPONSIBILITIES—
healthcare and financial affairs. First, we looked for ways to keep
Mardig active during the day. In Milwaukee, he was familiar with his
neighborhood and went on walks, shopped, did his banking, etc. Here
everything is spread out and my father was unfamiliar with the area.
He loved to read, so we ordered the newspaper for him. He read it and
magazines and books. After several days, he started growing increasingly stir-crazy. He wanted to do *something*! His nearly unquenchable
appetite for reading had hit even his saturation level.

I looked around for things to do. Living in a newer home, there
were limited opportunities for him to do what he loved—fix things.
We did have a couple of outdoor electrical outlets that were giving us
some problems. I asked him if he was willing to fix these. He said he
would and fixed them in one afternoon. This wasn't enough to keep
his mind active. He needed more.

Mardig looked in the paper for a job. I promised him I would help
him find a job. I seriously thought about him working at Wal-Mart
since they hire retirees. My father was warm, congenial, and personable. He would love it! As my mind brainstormed job opportunities
for him, I nearly forgot that he was impaired. Although slight at first,
his occasional bouts of disorientation could prove problematic at a *real*
job.

I looked at other options. Sally used to take her father to the local

Visiting Nurses Association's (VNA) Adult Day Care Center and high-ly recommended it. It kept her father's mind active and allowed him to socialize with others. At first, I didn't like the idea. It didn't make sense. After all, parents take their *kids* to day care. You don't take your *parents* to day care. At least this is what I thought. (There was so much I had to learn.)

Since Sally strongly urged me to consider day care, I called to inquire. Roberta, the administrator at the VNA, answered the tele-phone. After explaining my situation to her, she invited me to visit.

A day later and unannounced, I went to see what the center looked like. Roberta was not prepared for my visit. She was occupied with the family of one of the female participants who would no longer be attending day care due to her declining health. Her son and daughter-in-law were in Roberta's office making the necessary arrangements and saying their good-byes.

Despite this, Roberta graciously made time for me. She tried to contain her sadness while explaining that over a short period of time the participants became her family. She couldn't hold back tears as she said good-bye to this woman, to whom she had grown so attached. She apologized for her tears. I was moved by Roberta's genuine feel-ings for this woman and, as I was to discover, the other participants. Even though Mardig was not a participant yet, I imagined her feeling this way about him someday, when he could no longer attend adult day care.

While Roberta split her time between the family and me, I watched the participants. I was not prepared for what I saw. I wasn't used to seeing adults *babied*. I saw mostly older participants who were each given the same warmth and compassion one would give to a child. I tried to accept it, as this was yet another new experience for me. I would try to understand more later by asking Sally about it that evening. I needed to get some perspective on what I saw and what I was feeling. *Besides, my options were rather limited!*

On the other hand, I was embarrassed. *Brenda's father is going to day care.* What would others think? *Besides, what kind of daughter would take her father to day care? Why not let him stay at home, where she can care for him? Why have someone else take the responsibility? This sounds like the dilemma faced by working parents of preschoolers.*

And then there were those other thoughts. *How could my father possibly fit in? He wasn't this bad.*

After watching the participants and talking with Roberta for a while, my feelings of embarrassment began melting away. I watched the staff's compassion for these people. I started justifying the concerns in my mind. *At least my father would be treated with kindness. He would be treated gently. He would receive the attention he needed—more than I, one person, was able to give.*

But what about customized care? Mardig couldn't go to day care. He wanted to work!

I asked Roberta about customized care. I explained that my father had a sincere need to feel useful. He didn't just want to help out or volunteer. He wanted to go to work and earn some money. He was not ready to retire.

She asked how old my father was.

"Eighty-six," I answered.

She smiled and chuckled. She explained that her staff offered unique care for each participant. If a participant wanted to go to work, the staff not only welcomed him to work, but also gave him tasks to perform. If another wanted to go to school, they welcomed her to school, and gave her lessons.

I was amazed. "You really do this?" I asked. This was just the tip of the iceberg of all they did! Mardig's care requirements would be minimal compared to the undergarments they changed for the incontinent participants, the frequent and complicated doses of medicine they administered, and the many other unique demands they fulfilled.

"Yes, of course!" Roberta replied. "Otherwise, the participants wouldn't be happy."

"You mean, you learn what each person needs and then you deal with them in that way?"

"Yes. If someone wants to go to school, she goes to school. If your father wants to go to work, he comes to work. Each member of our

staff will refer to 'work' when speaking with your father," she emphasized.

This was certainly a plus in their favor. I liked this personal touch.
We spoke for about forty-five minutes, and I met a few other members
of her staff—Ellie, Tee, David, and Kathy—and a few of the participants.

I was getting used to the idea that even though Mardig seemed to
be in better shape than these participants, activity was important for
him. After all, I had businesses to run. I couldn't be occupied with him
twenty-four hours a day.

I told Roberta I'd give it a try. She gave me paperwork to complete
and to bring with me when I brought my father in.

I went home and discussed the idea with Mardig. I explained that
going to this place (I took care not to call it by name.) would be like
a job. It would be his initial training before he could move up into
higher-level responsibilities. He was thrilled. He said he'd try it. I filled
out the forms Roberta gave me.

Now I was stuck with my conscience. I had lied to my father. He
was not stupid. He would see the day care for what it was and then ask
me why I had taken him to a place where they made crafts, did busy-
work—and took frequent breaks.

*I remember visiting my father at the neighborhood factory he worked
at part-time in the mornings. I was between ten and thirteen years old.
It was summertime, when kids looked for different things to do since school
was out. I would walk about one mile, sometimes alone or with my sister,
to visit him at work. I would wait for the bell to ring, signaling break
time. When I wouldn't see him, I'd look inside the dimly lit factory and
be surprised to see him still working. Usually, one of his co-workers would
notice me and ask if I wanted to see my father. I'd eagerly nod and say,
"Yes!" He'd explain, "Oh, Marty? He's still working. He should be on
break, but he just keeps working. Wait and I'll get 'im for you."*

*While I waited, I'd be a little afraid of how my father would react,
since I was interrupting his work. Sometimes, I'd just walk up to the
machine he was working on and he'd look up with a big smile and say,*

"Oh, let me finish up. Wait for me outside and I'll come out and talk with you." (This was in the days before OSHA's regulations impacted this factory.) He'd come out and talk with me. Then, five minutes later, before the bell rang to signal people back to work, he'd say, "I have to get back to work. Thank you for visiting. Are you going home now?" I would be a little disappointed that he had cut our visit short to return to work before break time was over. After all, I had walked quite a distance. But that's the way he was.

I discussed the lie I had told my father with David. What would happen if Mardig saw through this charade and realized this was not a job and was just a place to socialize and stay active? Then again, he *worked* at home. He was always working on one thing or another, taking one machine apart, cleaning it, and then putting it back together. He was reorganizing his papers, taking care of his banking, organizing his tools, and working around the outside of the house. David and I decided to take the chance.

He would benefit from the socialization and the activities. Mardig had been a hermit for so long. During his last few months in Milwaukee, he spent most of his days at home, puttering with various fix-it items or trying to process his paperwork—except when he went grocery shopping and visited the bank. Still, we were concerned about lying to him. We slept restlessly that night. I worried about Mardig's reaction. I certainly did not want to offend him, or more importantly, lose his trust.

The following morning Mardig showered at my urging ("You want to be clean for your first day of work.") and put on the clothes I had selected for him. He was pleased that I made such a fuss over him.

He said, "Even Ma (referring to my mother) didn't fuss over me this much!" *Well, maybe she didn't during the last years of her life, but she certainly did while he was working. He was without a doubt the cleanest and best-dressed machinist at General Electric—his full-time job in the afternoons. He showered twice a day and my mother always made sure he had clean and pressed clothes to wear to work each day.*

We had breakfast and joked about his first day at a new job. I teased him and asked him to be good, that I didn't want any calls from his supervisor. He said he'd make me proud, because he knew my reputation was riding on this job referral. I was pleased he was looking forward to his new job, but I knew in my heart I had lied.

I drove him to *work* and the staff warmly welcomed him. After asking how he liked his coffee, a smiling staff member offered him a cup with plenty of cream and sugar. He was not typically a coffee drinker, yet he liked the sweet and creamy taste. He was taken by the warm reception. I handed the completed paperwork to Roberta, and she assured me there was nothing to worry about. "We'll take good care of your father," another staff member added.

I returned home, to peace and uninterrupted quiet. I immediately started to work. Soon the worries crept in. After one and a half hours of wondering and not being able to concentrate on my work, I called and asked how my father was doing. The staff member who answered the phone assured me he was doing great. She added that he was a hit with the ladies. *This was a side of my father I didn't know about!* My heart grew calmer knowing that he was fitting in. I was happy for him. There was, however, still a little nagging question about what he would say when I picked him up that afternoon. Since Mardig is the master diplomat, he wouldn't say anything to people at *work*. He would wait until he saw me.

That afternoon I went to pick Mardig up and to bring him home. He looked happy and was in a joyful mood. The staff expressed how much they had enjoyed him and asked if I would bring him in again the following day. I said I'd like to, but first I wanted to see how he would react that evening.

On the way home, Mardig expressed how much he enjoyed what he had done. He said if *that* was called work then work had changed a lot from when he worked at General Electric. *He hadn't seen through the charade!*

When David came home later, Mardig said the same thing to him. We were pleased. This meant that he would be around people, involved in a variety of activities, go out for walks, and most importantly, supervised by a caring staff. This also meant I would have six hours each day to accomplish my work.

～   ～

FOR THE MOST PART, THIS ROUTINE WORKED FINE. Mardig enjoyed day care and the activities it offered. I was told he particularly relished dancing with the ladies. Considering there were more ladies than men attending day care, he frequently danced with different partners. Since he was in such good physical shape, he'd dance every dance, tiring his partners who were many years his junior! I was happy for him.

Each afternoon when I picked him up, the staff told me what he had worked on that day. Sometimes, Mardig would bring home something he had created. He wouldn't think much of it and toss it aside, but I would treasure it like a proud parent. After all, my father had created it!

Mardig wandered at the adult day care, just as he had at home. Sometimes he wandered too much and was a challenge to the staff, particularly when he refused to return after walking outside. Once, when I was away on travel, he refused to return. The staff had to call David at work to help control Mardig. David left immediately and made the two-hour drive from his office to the day care center just to bring Mardig home.

Despite the challenges, adult day care gave my father many opportunities to socialize, to remain active, to think, to smile, to laugh, and to do all the things he deserved to do.

With adult day care, I thought I could reasonably anticipate a routine in Mardig's schedule. After I brought him home, he'd get the mail and then read magazines until David came home about 6:00 p.m. Then we'd eat dinner. We would talk for a while, read, or watch television. Mardig preferred to go to bed early, about 8:30 p.m. David and I would stay up and do housework or read the mail.

I started adapting to my father's schedule. David would rise at 4:15 a.m. to make the long drive to Los Angeles. I would get up an hour later to get some work done before my father woke up. Mardig would sometimes get up and come into my office to talk. I used to encourage him to go back to bed so that he would be well rested for work. Usually he did. Then I would continue working until 6:30 a.m., when I went into his room to wake him.

As the weeks passed, Mardig began to refuse to return to bed after he'd wake early in the morning. He'd come into my home office, fully dressed and ready to leave for *work*. Each morning, I tried to talk him into going back to bed. He wouldn't. I didn't know what to do.

One morning I closed the door to my office, hoping he wouldn't notice me. He didn't bother me that morning. I heard him walk around, open the refrigerator door, and then return to his room. I got up from my chair, quietly opened my door, and peered down the hallway toward his room. I tiptoed to the kitchen to see if he had closed the refrigerator door tightly. Everything looked fine. I noticed a candy wrapper on the counter and saw that a few pieces of candy were missing from the candy bowl.

I quietly tiptoed toward his room. He had left his door slightly ajar. From the small opening, I saw him sitting in the rocking chair with his back turned to me. I wasn't sure whether he was sleeping or not. Curiosity got the better of me, so I slowly opened the door, uncertain whether it would creak and he would hear me. It didn't. Since he couldn't hear well, I was able to sneak right beside him. His eyes were closed. Three crumbled up candy wrappers were on the floor, and one of David's engineering books rested on his lap. On one of the bookshelves, within easy reach, was a partially filled glass of milk. Despite the urge to wake him and help him back to bed, where he would be more comfortable, I left him be and went back into my office and closed the door.

I thought about how sore his neck and back would probably be from sleeping in the chair. He never complained. After about two hours, he knocked on my door. I stopped what I was doing to make breakfast. We talked until it was time for me to take him to *work*.

I tried this the next morning. It worked. I tried it again. It worked. It is said, if something works, don't change it.

Sometimes I could work for an hour and a half before Mardig would knock on my office door. He was polite. Most often he would knock before entering.

At first, I would help him shower every other morning and get dressed, which was a major struggle in itself. Then I would prepare breakfast and take him to the Adult Day Care Center.

Our morning ritual did not, however, always go smoothly.

Chapter 7

"WHERE'S MY SHOES?"

*L*IVING WITH OTHER PEOPLE CAN PRESENT CHALLENGES. David and I ask our guests to take off their shoes in the foyer before entering our home. This way our carpets stay clean longer, and if we want to sit or lie down on the floor, we don't have to worry about what is tracked in off the street. On the other hand, Mardig, a product of the depression, believed that *a man needs to wear his shoes.*

This was fine and well. We bought him a pair of suede slippers. They weren't good enough. He was used to heavy leather shoes with thick leather soles. And so, the irritations began...

"Mardig, please don't wear your shoes in the house."

"Why?"

"Because we don't wear shoes in the house. It keeps the carpet cleaner."

"My shoes are not dirty. See?" he says as he turns up the soles of his shoes to prove his point.

"Yes, I see. But you don't know where they've been. We like to sit and lie on the floor without worrying about germs."

Mardig was never one to worry about germs. "A little germ won't hurt anyone," he'd tease my mother when she would remind him to wash his hands.

We went around and around. David and I began to realize this wasn't going anywhere.

What's the big deal? All we need to do is get the carpets cleaned. Oh, but this requires calling someone, setting time aside to have them come in and clean, moving furniture, putting those little foil pieces under the legs of tables, dressers, couches, etc., waiting for the carpet to dry...we didn't have time for this! My father was going to cooperate on this one thing!

We had to come up with a plan. We would wait until Mardig took his shoes off before going to bed. We would then hide his shoes. We would only give him his shoes before he went outside.

When Mardig went to bed that night, we went in to say good night, then discreetly stooped down, plucked his shoes from where they were neatly lined up under the foot of his bed, and pirouetted right out of there without his realizing what had happened.

That night, Mardig awoke, got dressed, and couldn't find his shoes. He came into our bedroom. And it began...those three words which would ring terror in our minds, *"Where's my shoes?"*

"Why...? Do you need them?"

"Yes. I'm going to work?"

"At *this* time?"

"I don't want to be late."

"You won't be. You're at least six hours early."

"I am?"

"Yes. You don't start work until eight."

"What time is it?"

"It's one-thirty in the morning."

"Oh, well, then *where's my shoes?* I don't want to be late."

Since David had more than a two-hour commute ahead of him in a little over three hours, I got up and took Mardig to his room to persuade him to go to sleep. After a half hour and a promise that I would wake him in time so that he wouldn't be late for *work*, Mardig undressed and went back to sleep.

Ahhh. Got away with that one. We didn't even have to tell him where his shoes were.

The next morning at 3:00 a.m. I heard, *"Where's my shoes?"*

I was sound asleep and awoke to David talking with Mardig in our bedroom.

~ ~

THIS HAD BECOME THE NEWEST, *VERY EARLY* MORNING RITUAL. Mardig would wake at any hour of the night and wander the house looking for someone…anyone. He would finally make his way into our bedroom. We would wake up after hearing him shuffle about. Parents know the feeling of being able to hear the slightest sounds their children make. Well, it was no different for us. We had made the decision to *adopt* my father and had taken on the role of parents.

Some mornings he would come into our bedroom and feel the walls for a light switch. After being surprised with a sudden bright light several predawn mornings in a row, we disconnected the wall switch from the light. *Even the sun takes time unveiling all of its brightness in the morning!*

In the past Mardig had used a flashlight. But he had taken it apart and put it together so many times that pieces were missing. This was a good thing, because having a flashlight shined in our faces in the wee hours of the morning was not exactly pleasant.

Since he didn't have any light, Mardig would navigate by feeling the walls, furniture, anything. As he approached our bed, we would lie still, even as he felt the bed and our bodies. This was a very weird sensation for both of us. *Here is Brenda's father feeling her and her husband in bed.* We were hoping Mardig wouldn't find anything or anyone and then go back to bed. This was not to be. He would get scared and start calling our names. Our hearts softened. We'd get up and encourage him to go back to bed. *Is this any different than caring for a frightened child?*

Weeks later, utterly exhausted, I talked with Sally. She was fortunate. Her father did not wander like Mardig. She recommended that we lock our bedroom door. David and I preferred to sleep with our bedroom door open. We had to adapt. We not only had to close it, but lock it as well. *But what about my father? Wouldn't this prove too traumatic for him?* When I raised these issues, Sally reminded me that David and I were running out of energy because we weren't getting enough sleep. She assured us that our ears would pick up the important sounds and this may be a way of discouraging Mardig from being up at night.

We tried it. We didn't sleep well the first night because we worried about how Mardig would fare. Mardig slept the entire night, except to go to the bathroom.

The second night he tried the door to our bedroom. He jiggled the doorknob. When it didn't open, we heard him walk away. Just as we drifted off to sleep, we heard the doorknob jiggle again. The constant jiggling throughout the night kept us awake. We lay silently and safely on the other side of that door, feeling *small* because we were hiding from my father and contributing to his discomfort.

Sadly, this is what we had to do for our sanity and rest. *But were we really getting any rest?* We heard him walk toward the living room. The following morning we found him sleeping on the recliner. He was wearing a jacket, pajamas, and slippers. He looked so innocent, so peaceful, like a child. I felt sorry for him because he had lost his sense of time.

Other nights we'd hear the creak of the front door to the house as he tried to leave. We have security screen doors that lock with a key. Mardig couldn't get out. After trying for some time, he'd return and jiggle the doorknob to our bedroom.

One night we heard noises in the utility room. We weren't sure what we were hearing so, despite exhaustion, I got up and quietly opened our bedroom door to look. I was shocked at what I saw. He was trying to remove the hinges on the door to the garage! I walked closer to see what kind of *tools* Mardig was using—scissors, nail clippers, and a piece of wood.

These nighttime explorations were wearing us down. Yet, our consciences were also preventing us from sleeping soundly. This was no way to treat another human being. *Children grow out of this and sleep through the night. With Alzheimer's, there is no growth, it only goes downhill.* We tried to rationalize our behavior. Nothing helped. We knew we weren't behaving in a totally caring manner. A parent would get up and comfort his/her child. Yet, trying to ignore him when he wasn't in any danger was the only way we could cope.

~   ~

"WHAT DO YOU MEAN?" David tried to delay answering my father's question.

"Someone has taken my shoes," Mardig clarified.

"We have them," I volunteered, opting for honesty.

"Why?"

"Because we don't want you wearing them in the house," I replied.

"Why did you take my shoes?" my father insisted.

"Because you wear them in the house," David answered firmly.

"Where are my shoes?"

"We have them," I said.

"They are *my* shoes," he emphasized.

"Yes, I know they are yours. And you will get them when you need to leave the house," I added.

"I'm leaving *now*!"

"At three in the morning?" David asked.

"That doesn't matter. I want *my* shoes."

~   ~

THAT EVENING, AFTER DINNER, MARDIG SURPRISED US WITH HIS REAC-
tion. He looked genuinely puzzled and then spoke slowly, as if thinking aloud. "You know, I take my shoes off and put them under the
bed, and then they disappear. Do you know where they are?"

"Yes, we have them."

"*You* have them?" he asked, surprised.

"Yes."

He chuckled and then added, "Why do *you* need my shoes?"

We didn't know whether he was being a diplomat by humoring us
or whether he was genuinely curious. It was hard to tell if this was him
or the disease talking.

~   ~

MORNINGS AND EVENINGS, EVERY DAY, MY FATHER WOULD ASK,
"Where's my shoes?" These three words, asked so often and at so
many inopportune times, caused David and me so much agony.

We even had to search for them. Mardig caught on relatively quickly and began hiding his shoes from us! It was a challenge to see who could hide Mardig's shoes from the other. First, he pushed them further under his bed. We found and removed them. Then they were behind the rocker by the bookshelf. It took a little doing, but we found and removed them. Then they were in the closet. It took a while but we found them…behind some boxes in the closet…behind the doors of the bookshelf. (This last hiding place required repeated visits to his room while one of us distracted him and the other looked.) Another time, he placed them in an obvious location. The only problem was, we didn't realize it until after we had searched the house on and off for a of couple hours. He had left his shoes in the breezeway, where he had taken them off earlier. *Wait a minute…he tricked us! David's shoes were missing!*

～ ～

IN TALKING WITH OTHERS, WE'VE LEARNED THAT THERE IS USUALLY ONE behavior that really bugs a caregiver—no, make that, *gnaws* at a caregiver's nerves. For each of us, it's something different.

Mardig would leave his used toothpicks in all kinds of places—on his bathroom counter, on the bookshelves, propped in books, on the stereo, on the kitchen counter, behind the stereo, in the computer's disk drive slot, and on the recliner (we found one by sitting down on it). We could deal with this habit. Even the bubblegum stuck to his nightstand or on the external hard drive was tolerable. None of these things annoyed us as much as that incessant question, "Where's my shoes?"

We had made the choice to take on this responsibility. There could be no regrets.

Chapter 8

MEDICAL EVALUATION & DRUG STUDY

W ITH EVERYTHING ELSE GOING ON, I made it a priority to schedule a medical evaluation for Mardig. Roberta and one of her staff members highly recommended the Granada Hills Community Hospital's CARE (Center for Aging Research and Evaluation). I called and left a message. When a woman named Bert returned my call, I explained my desire to have my father evaluated by specialists before I departed on a business trip. We had just brought Mardig to California and I wanted to make sure he was not facing any immediate health problems. Bert scheduled the initial evaluation one week later.

Marlene Harrison, Director of CARE, called a few days later to ask questions as part of the pre-visit assessment. I felt a little uneasy answering medical-related questions on behalf of my father. It was difficult getting used to being responsible for another adult—one whose medical history was only beginning to unfold before my eyes.

꙳   ꙳

AFTER A ONE-HOUR DRIVE TO THE SAN FERNANDO VALLEY (north of Los Angeles) and signing lots of paperwork, I found the staff at CARE to be warm and thoughtful with my father. He was pleased with the attention. I could see the CARE staff knew what they were doing and felt confident that my father would receive a thorough evaluation.

For the first two and a half hours his vital signs (blood pressure, pulse, temperature, height, weight) were checked. He gave blood and urine samples, and he was given a mental test to evaluate his aware-ness and recall. He was also seen by Dr. Weinberg, a neurologist who specializes in dementia. During the two following visits, Mardig received every test imaginable. Among them were a chest X-ray (a matter of procedure since he did not have a recent one on record), an EEG, and an EKG.

He also received one of the most informative verbal evaluations I've seen—a speech/language/cognitive/memory evaluation. Marlys Meckler went well beyond her role as a speech pathologist and offered many useful suggestions for my father's care.

For example, she suggested that David and I label each door in the house to make it easier for my father to orient himself. We made huge labels with three-inch letters on the computer and pasted them to each door—OUTSIDE; MARDIG'S ROOM; BRENDA'S OFFICE; DAVID'S & BRENDA'S BEDROOM; GARAGE DOOR. Marlys suggested that we establish eye contact and gently touch Mardig to get his attention. She encouraged us to have him use his hearing aid (she explained how to use it). She said sharing photos of family members would better orient him (we created a photo album). Regarding appointments, Marlys suggested that we tell him shortly before he is ready to go. Finally, she advised we break all activities into simple steps: "Put on your shirt." "Here are your pants." "Put on your jacket." "Remember your glasses."

Mardig enjoyed all the attention he was getting. On our return trips he would comment upon how fortunate he was for all the trou-ble I was going through just for him.

During one of the earlier visits with CARE, Dr. Weinberg (a mild-mannered and soft-spoken man) recommended Mardig see a podia-trist for the fungal infection on his toes and toenails; that he have an eye exam before Alzheimer's progressed so far that he couldn't com-municate the quality of images for his eye exam (e.g., "Which can you see better, this or this?"); and that he see a dermatologist for the skin sores we noticed when we saw him scratching his legs. I made these appointments immediately upon my return from my business trip. Additionally, I scheduled a dental appointment for him. Within one month Mardig was seen by most of the doctors and specialists.

When I asked Marlene for the results of the evaluation, she explained that CARE uses a team concept where a gerontological registered nurse, medical doctor, psychologist, pharmacist, and other representatives meet to discuss each patient's case. Out of this meeting comes a comprehensive report. In this day of rush-rush assembly-line care (not while you're waiting, but once you're seen by the doctor), I was surprised to see so much time dedicated to my father.

When all was finished I received approximately twenty pages of single spaced, typed reports and an in-person briefing on Mardig that included: elaborate background history, social and family history, physical and neurological examinations, and overall comments. I was impressed. At least we knew Mardig's health was good and that there were no urgent health issues that required immediate attention.

Each time I drove my father the fifty-two miles to CARE, I felt like the mother of a child. It was amazing. I had taken Mardig to the doctor more often than I had gone myself. I was making sure every detail of his total healthcare was assessed and recorded.

◡   ◠

ONLY THREE MONTHS AFTER MARDIG MOVED TO CALIFORNIA, in December 1996, we decided to enroll him in a drug study. The drug, donepezil hydrochloride (Aricept®), had just been approved by the FDA and was still undergoing research to gain additional data on its effectiveness. All study participants would receive the actual drug in five or ten milligram doses.

David and I spoke with Dr. Jacobs, the doctor who was conducting the study, and with Dr. Weinberg, who initially examined Mardig. We asked many questions about Aricept® and read everything we could find on the drug.

In order to be accepted in the study, Mardig had a number of hurdles to cross first. We set an appointment to have him go through an initial screening (vitals and mental testing) and a physical exam. Once he passed these tests, we set an appointment for his baseline exam.

We took the time to get Mardig in the drug study for two reasons. First, the drug might actually help him get better. He had been declining during the past few weeks and we hoped he could improve enough to manage his own affairs. His financial affairs had taken far more time than we ever anticipated. *He may even be able to move back to his home!* This was really our fantasy. Kim Wilms, the drug study coordinator, assured us that no such improvement had been documented.

Second, the Aricept® study would place him under the intense scrutiny of a doctor. This would certainly be an advantage toward the quality of his care since Pfizer and Eisai, the pharmaceutical companies sponsoring the study, and the FDA had special requirements.

I asked more questions of Dr. Jacobs, an uncommonly attired doctor, because I wanted to be sure I was making the right decision on my father's behalf. It took me time to get used to a doctor who donned cowboy gear—a loose denim shirt unbuttoned at the collar, tight-fitting jeans with a belt and the requisite oversized buckle, finished off with cowboy boots. I later learned that this personable and knowledgeable doctor transported himself to and from work on a motorcycle. *My father is about to go on a drug study with a motorcycle riding cowboy!*

Mardig seemed unfazed by Dr. Jacobs' attire, never saying a word about it. I signed the study contract and agreed to provide CARE with regular reports of Mardig's condition.

ᵕ   ᵎ

ON DECEMBER 18, I STARTED KEEPING A DAILY JOURNAL of Mardig for the study. I jotted notes whenever I could. This lasted for a little over a month.

What follows is most of my journal (in unedited form).

Wednesday, December 18, 1996
Took Mardig to CARE. A funny thing happened during Mardig's mental evaluation. Mardig was asked to name as

many words as he could that begin with "s." Mardig's first word, "sex." In contrast to his condition, the number of three syllable words he effortlessly listed proved that all the years he had spent reading had served him well. Accepted into drug study. Took first pill (5 mg) at 5:10 p.m. while still at CARE.

Went to dinner in North Hollywood (to celebrate and to avoid traffic going home). After seeing the "Hollywood" street sign, Mardig could not believe "Hollywood" was in Chicago. He suggested spending the night in a hotel. After dinner, he didn't want to drive a long time. (He probably thought we were farther away than we were.) Arrived home at 10:00 p.m. ...amazed at how all his stuff was here...how it looked the same. Wanted to leave...got mean...said unkind things.

Thursday, December 19, 1996
8:00 a.m. Talked about his terrible dream last night.

Friday, December 20, 1996
Irritated...came into my office twice within five minutes asking where he can go for a haircut. Couldn't hear my answer. Wouldn't wear hearing aid. Wanted shoes.

Saturday, December 21, 1996
Agitated. Incident where he wore shoes in the house and refused to take them off.

Went out in backyard...looked around for something? Came inside and then went out a second time and was gone! David took his cell phone and went on foot to find him. Followed him at a distance for 40 minutes...Mardig asked strangers where he lived...tried to evade David.

I came later with the car and picked up David. Driving alongside while Mardig was walking, we tried to persuade him to come into the car. He refused. We backed-off awhile and then started losing patience tracking him from a comfortable distance. Once he reached the busy street we decided to use force, if necessary, to get him in the car. We were afraid of him walking alone on a busy street. My adrenaline rushing, I stopped the car in the far right lane of the six-lane street. I turned on the hazard lights and left it running. As Mardig's POA, I told David to do whatever it took to get him in the car. I didn't want any battery charges to emerge later because a son-in-law used physical force. *This was like kidnapping. We've seen it on television when a van pulls up next to a play-ground, a person comes out, snatches a child, and then the van speeds away.* We were afraid, shaking, wondering what we would say if someone saw us and interfered. We had to act fast.

David and I got on each side of Mardig, and lifted him up from under his arms and carried him kicking and screaming a few yards to the car. I turned him around to face me and tried to push him into the backseat of the car. He wouldn't lower his head. Remembering something I'd seen on TV, I tried to get him to bend by applying pressure to his stomach. It worked, he bent and then screamed that his head was hitting the car. It wasn't, my hand was on top of his head with two inches to spare. Once we got him inside the car, I asked David to sit in the backseat with him. I drove with Mardig ranting and raving that kidnapping is against the law and that he could have us arrested for hurting him. I told him we were doing this for his own good. I told him that I would take him to the sheriff's sta-tion so he could file a report if he really believed we did wrong. He continued complaining, so I drove to the station and asked him if he wanted to get out and file a report. He hesitated. I volunteered to come inside with him. He refused to go inside. He said it would get us in trouble and that he didn't want to hurt us. *Phew!*

After I pulled the car into the attached garage and closed the door, I had to cajole him back into the house. He was con-cerned about losing face if he came into house. David, who was shaken by this whole experience, had already gone inside. I tried to encourage my father. Later, and with a lot of prompting, he came in, ate some snacks, and then played a game of backgammon. I knew things were starting to turn for the better, when he said, "My brain is too small to learn such a complex game!"

Sunday, December 22, 1996
Some obstinateness and appearance of depression. Stayed in his room. We brought him his paper and warm chocolate milk. He came out later and helped us make breakfast by frying the bacon. We discussed finances after breakfast...he wanted to strategize how to keep his finances a secret..."just you and me need to know," he said to me. Insisted on finding his wallet before we left to go shopping. We looked for 20 minutes. He forgot what he was looking for.

Monday, December 23, 1996 (David's notes)
Irritated about Alzheimer's bracelet. Kept trying to take it off. Always speaks of his shoes being taken. Seemed depressed in evening.

Wednesday, December 25, 1996 (David's notes)
Got up. Wanted his shoes in order to leave to do his job. Kept insisting that he had to leave. Wanted to leave wearing his pajamas. Was very irritated in the morning before we left. We drove a friend to the Burbank airport and then went to Oxnard to see the ocean and walk on the beach. He was pleasant the rest of the day. We opened gifts in the evening while Brenda and I took turns videotaping it. Afterward, we watched a videotape from Thanksgiving in Las Vegas, our day in Oxnard at the ocean, and all of us opening our gifts. He recognized himself on TV!

Thursday, December 26, 1996 (David's notes)
He ate candy at 5:30 a.m. I found the bag in the middle of the living room floor. He was so charged, he wanted to leave right away and go to work. He kept trying to leave the house. I took him to the Adult Day Care Center at 8:15.

He didn't want dinner when we came home. He went to bed at 6:30 p.m.—wanted to be ready for tomorrow.

(Brenda's notes)

Woke up at 10:40 p.m. and wanted to know when we were to leave...disoriented as to time of day...thought it was day-time...lost shaver...hid it in box in closet...didn't believe he did this. Wanted to lock things up so "they don't take and use them."

Friday, December 27, 1996 (David's notes)

Easy to deal with in the morning. Went to dermatologist. Appeared nervous. Removed hearing aid before doctor walked in room. Said doctor should talk loudly so we can get our money's worth(??)

Saturday, December 28, 1996 (David's notes)

Woke up when heard him trying to leave. First question in the morning, "Where's my shoes?" After we convinced him that he wasn't going anywhere, he settled down. This convincing took 1 1/2 hours. We went for a three-mile walk in the afternoon. He was cooperative. It appears that parts of his memory are coming back. When asked, he remembered he had three children, knew his home address in Milwaukee, knew [Brenda's sister's] address, and he mentioned these things without hesitation. He knew these things in his slightly irritated state. It could be that he knew these things just because he was mentally alert for some reason (up and down days), or the drug might be working. He also had a severe case of "Sundowner's syndrome." He insisted that he had to go home and couldn't understand that this was home. He finally gave in but was a bit depressed because he started to realize he was confused as to where he was. His cognitive abilities seem to be improving—he has figured out how to open the large garage door (by pushing the button along the side of the doorway). He also figured out how to get out of the backyard—we think he broke the latch on the gate. I may be reading into it. But these are the things that are different.

Sunday, December 29, 1996 (David's notes)
Read Sunday paper.

Monday, December 30, 1996
Very cooperative. Aricept® seems to be working. Had #3 tooth pulled (due to infection and nerve damage) at about 3:00 p.m. He was not aware that this would happen until about 30 minutes before. He was very apprehensive about it and did not really like the whole situation. Afterward, he stopped bleeding and felt no pain. He is on penicillin 4 times a day. I have Tylenol #3 in case he needs it, but he has felt nothing. Went to bed about 8:30.

Tuesday, December 31, 1996 (David's notes)
Very cooperative and pleasant. It appears that his cognitive abilities are improving—he was very interested in reading a story in *Reader's Digest*—he could even tell a little what the story was about. He is more able to maintain the thread of the conversation. His appetite seems to be increasing.

Went to bed about 8:00 p.m. and woke up at 12:00 a.m., got dressed and wanted to leave to go to work—could not understand the time—was irritated because we would not give him his shoes. Wanted to eat. We prepared a snack for him and then we went to bed. He stayed up for a while.

Wednesday, January 1, 1997
For the first time in a long time (nearly four months) Mardig was able to sit and focus on one thing for two and a half hours. He watched the colorful floats in the Rose Bowl Parade on TV. He was mesmerized! Then we took him to Mount Wilson overlooking Pasadena. He seemed to handle the altitude (5600') quite well, including the three and a half narrow staircases up to the 100-inch Mt. Wilson telescope. We walked for quite a

bit in what turned out to be a cold drizzly day and he fared well. He was initially afraid as we were driving up the winding mountain road... "Slow down!" he'd yell, a little irritated. "Keep your eye on the road!"

Afterward, he was happy we made the trip. "This was really worth it!" he said.

Thursday, January 2, 1997

Mardig's cognitive ability appears to have declined. On the way home from day care he asked, "Where's Ma?" He hadn't asked this in awhile. He seemed surprised and unaware of his mother and mine (his wife) not being alive. He couldn't even picture their faces he said. I showed him their pictures when we got home. He then asked if there was anyone else like me (i.e., siblings) here. He laughed when I explained they were in Milwaukee and we were in California. He laughed again when I reminded him we're in California.

I gave him a book to read, *Ring Around the Moon*, by Lois Erisey Poole, a local author. He read a few pages then set it aside with the comment, "I will digest it later."

Friday, January 3, 1997

"Where's my shoes?" Ahh...welcome to the mornings with Mardig...every morning...rare not to hear this question.

Evening...Mardig watched TV. He didn't listen to the content so much as the *meta-content* (how the speaker was delivering the message, his nationality, and his persuasiveness). When I asked him about the content he said he missed the beginning so he won't bother with the rest...he'll wait until later to digest it. Later and after closing his eyes awhile, he asked if this was the same speaker he was watching earlier. He often watched TV like this. It was almost as if interpreting the content was too difficult and so he commented on what he could see and the inflections he could hear.

Tuesday, January 7, 1997

It appears Mardig is experiencing more peaks and valleys. He seemed more alert and aware for two days and, the other two days he seemed disoriented and confused.

Thursday, January 16, 1997

Mardig caught the flu Monday...was difficult at the Day Care Center...when he came home he had 102° temp. Gave him Tylenol to bring down fever. Called CARE to report per requirements for participation in drug study.

Mardig started having bouts of incontinence—urinated on the floor in front of the toilet; urinated in his pants—five incidents thus far.

Took Mardig to our doctor with a 101.5° fever. Didn't want to take any chances. Doctor prescribed antibiotic for partially infected (greenish) mucous.

Monday, January 20, 1997 (David's notes)

Kept asking "Where's the flashlight?" while he was holding one. When I told him he had one in his hand, he said "Yeah, but where's the flashlight?" Really confused.

Tuesday, January 21, 1997

Mardig seems to have declined in his ability to tell time. Does not know day from night by looking at the clock. His focus has also declined. It may also be that we are unable to keep on top of all his needs. We ask him to do one thing, and he does another. "Put in your hearing aid." He says okay and goes to his room and gets a toothpick.

There's a song he hums...used to hum it when he felt good. Now he hums it in order to feel good or hold onto a memory. We wish we could buy a recording of it, but we're not sure of the name. One friend thought it was called, *Good Night Irene*. We were unable to find this at the local music store.

A bit ornery—turns off hearing aid and then expects to converse. Can't hear and says, "Huh?"

(David's notes)

No longer concerned about taxes—I don't think he knows or understands what taxes are—just signed papers without reading—unusual for him.

Thursday, January 23, 1997

8:30 a.m. After growing frustrations, cleaning up the mess due to his incontinence, his refusal to listen, and getting just plain exhausted keeping on top of everything, I had a discussion with Mardig regarding not wearing his shoes in the house, his self-centeredness, etc.

"Let me be until I die," he replied at my expressions of frustration.

Stubborn. Won't wear hearing aid. ("If you care for me you'll talk louder.")

Took him to adult day care.

When I picked him up in the afternoon, he said he liked the warmth of the car. He said he felt chilled during the day. Refused to get out of the car when we came home. Sat in car while it was parked in garage. When I came out into the garage five minutes later, he said he wanted to sleep in car. I tried to convince him to come in but he wouldn't. I went back inside and then came out again, five minutes later. This time he motioned with his hand for me to go away. I could hear him humming a different tune!

We're getting less patient in dealing with him...getting tired.

One of the requirements of the drug study was a series of follow-up visits to monitor Mardig's condition while on Aricept®. One of these appointments was scheduled during a week in February when David and I would be out of town. Kim volunteered to drive the fifty-two miles to see my father.

On March 12th I brought Mardig to CARE for his last follow-up visit. I scrawled the following notes on three pieces of paper.

Wednesday, March 12, 1997

Trip down...Asked questions all the way down...one after another...like a child...chattering...asking same question ("Are you going to a particular place?") within five minutes of saying "Okay," to my answer.

Since we arrived early, I debated whether to go into a public place with him. Toured the hilly areas just west of Balboa Blvd. in the San Fernando Valley. I was told that some of this real estate sold in the range of $250,000 (smaller homes) to over $1,000,000 (larger homes with more land). He was amazed at the cost! We still had more time so we went to Circuit City to look for a palm-sized television. My father started humming very loudly. I felt self-conscious about my demented father's behavior amidst all the youth in this store. So I took his arm and we quickly exited.

He is now sitting next to me in an office here at GHCH—CARE...humming and talking loudly...then pleading jokingly, "I wanna go home." Now reading a magazine...occupied...quiet.

Into my realm of awareness enters the sound of a man's voice asking, "Who am I here to see?" A woman answers. He repeats her answer, "Dr. Jacobs?" Then I hear, "Oh, okay." All is quiet and then I hear the question again, "Who am I here to see?" This happens several times. Must be the disease.

Dr. Jacobs reviewed notes...he says my father has moderate Alzheimer's—in the middle stage of Alzheimer's.

He then gave Mardig a little test. He drew a circle and told him it was a clock. He asked Mardig to write in the numbers of the clock. My father drew four little hash marks. Each was spaced equa-distant from the other—one at the 12:00 spot, another at 3:00, and the other two at 6:00 and 9:00. *This was a good start. He's going to do just fine!* He paused for a moment and then wrote the number "1" at the 10:00 position and ended with "3" at the 11:30 position. He then wrote the number 12 at the 1:00 position and ended with the number "2" at the 2:30 position. *What could he possibly be thinking?* The doctor asked if there was anything more. Mardig wrote the number "6" at the 5:00 position and then the numbers "7" through "10" were squeezed in the space occupied from 6:30 to 8:30.

Amazing. I sat quietly as I always did while he was being tested. My desire to help him was tempered by how privileged I felt to be able to stay in the room during these evaluations.

After the doctor finished, Aris, a staff member, came in with a green booklet, the same one used during Mardig's previous visits during this drug study, and asked him the same questions she had asked before. These questions will give her a sense of his awareness of time and location. She said this was the *Mini-Mental State Exam.*

"What is today's date?" she asked.

"I don't care."

"What is...year?"

"Nineteen fifty-seven."

"Can you tell me what season it is?"

"Approaching winter."

"What country are we in?"

"We're in Russia."

"What state...?"

"Used to be Wisconsin," my father said, nervously laughing.

"...city?"

"Used to be Milwaukee, when I was small."

"What building are we in?"

"It's a federal item."

"What floor are we on?"

"First floor."

Throughout this question and answer period, Mardig repeatedly stopped her and asked questions. When he did not know the answer to one of her questions, he'd explain why he didn't know. This ten-minute test stretched out to 20 minutes.

Next, she asked him to spell "WORLD." He managed this easily. Then she asked him to spell "WORLD" backward. This is what he said, "D L R O" and then after pausing for a moment, he added, "L D."

She asked him to do a few more things.

"Close your eyes, Mr. Avadian."

He looked directly at her and said, "Close your eyes."

She repeated the request.

He covered his eyes. He sat there, with each hand covering one eye, until she told him he could open his eyes.

She asked him to write a sentence on a blank sheet of paper. The sentence could be anything that came to his mind.

He wrote, "This teacher's too critical." During his last visit, he wrote that he hoped he was giving the right answers. During an earlier visit he wrote, "I hope this does some good." On another visit he wrote a paragraph about not understanding why he was being evaluated.

She asked him to copy two pentagons already printed on another page in the book. Previously, he would effortlessly reproduce the geometric designs. This time Mardig could not easily reproduce them.

I was sad that my father was declining in his ability. When he first came in for the initial screening on December 18, he received a rating of 21. A perfect score is 30. One week later, during the baseline exam for the study, he scored 17. Four weeks later, 16. Eight weeks later, 19. On this occasion, he scored a 14.

After this testing Mardig was removed from the drug study because he no longer qualified. We realized Aricept® had delayed his decline. We had such strong expectations that my father would improve enough to live his dreams, the dreams he kept putting off. We failed to see that Aricept® had helped him remain level. Once off of the drug the disease continued its course. I would have to accept what was, if I was to enjoy whatever time was left with my father.

Chapter 9

MONEY, MONEY, MONEY

Once my father's health needs were being taken care of, I set out to get his financial affairs in order.

When David and I initially agreed to care for Mardig and handle his affairs, we were aware he owned General Electric stock and U.S. Savings Bonds. We also knew of two checking and savings accounts, in addition to one or two Certificates of Deposit. At best, we figured Mardig was worth $200,000.

This would be easy. Mardig had granted me power of attorney over his two bank accounts. All I would have to do is transfer all of his finances so we could handle his affairs in California. David and I figured the sooner we took care of his affairs the sooner we'd be able to get back to our own business while dealing with Mardig's day-to-day care.

"**W**HAT DO I HAVE?"

While I was in Milwaukee in March 1996, my father invited me to go with him to the bank. He said he needed to take care of a few things. His bank was a half-mile away, and he said he wanted to walk for exercise. I said I'd accompany him. It would be a good opportunity for us to be outdoors. As it turned out, at nearly fifty years his junior, I could barely keep up with his rapid pace, much less carry on a conversation without getting out of breath.

I felt funny standing by while he did his banking. My parents had kept their financial affairs private. When I applied for a financial aid grant to attend the University of Wisconsin-Milwaukee, they refused to complete the paperwork because they didn't want anyone to know what they had in the bank. So, there I stood, trying not to look involved, thinking about my childhood.

My thoughts were interrupted when I overheard the customer service representative curtly tell Mardig, "Mr. Avadian, you came here two days ago asking for that information."

"Well, now I want it," Mardig said calmly.

"We gave you a printout of what you have!"

I wondered if she was being unnecessarily rude, so I started to pay attention. I stepped closer to Mardig and asked him what he needed. He looked at me briefly and then looked back at the woman and demanded, "I want to know what I have in my accounts."

Flustered, she relented and said, "Okay, I'll give you another printout."

Having succeeded, he looked at me with glee. I asked him what he was trying to do. He explained that he didn't want the bank to forget about his money so he had to keep track of what he owned.

The next moment, Mardig shifted his focus to some brochures. I used his inattentiveness to introduce myself to the representative and to ask what was going on.

She apologized for her behavior and said that Mardig would come to the bank three times a week asking about his money.

I was surprised. I couldn't believe he was so preoccupied with his accounts. "Really?" I asked.

"Yes," she said looking down.

"Why?"

"He forgets," she said.

"Wow, that must get kind of irritating," I added.

She looked up with a smile and asked, "You're his daughter?"

"Yes, I am." I stood a little taller.

"Well, you should see about him giving you power of attorney so you can help him with his finances."

"What?"

She explained that a POA would give me authority to handle his accounts. Given my childhood experiences, my heart raced with excitement. *I couldn't believe this was happening!* I calmed myself and said I would think about it because I had a sister and brother who might want to be involved.

I walked away feeling a sense of vindication. I had been invited to enter the secret domain of my father's finances. WOW, was I tickled!

~:   ~

DAYS LATER, MARDIG ASKED ME TO HELP HIM WITH HIS FINANCES. He said, "Talk with the bank and I will coach you to make sure they don't cheat us." He stood by proudly as I became his right arm and got what he wanted from the bank. Then he said, "Let's go to the other bank. Now I want you to ask for...."

It was on such an occasion that he granted me POA at one of his banks. If I recall, it was a matter of signing a little form. Yet, I was afraid. I had repeatedly asked my sister and brother to be involved in Mardig's care and affairs. They didn't respond. I felt alone.

Despite this, I had enough foresight to avoid unnecessary complications. I asked Mardig to grant me POA at the other bank. He declined. I thought, "It's his business."

Five months later, when I saw him in August, he asked me to be his POA at his other bank. He said he liked how I was keeping track of his papers. He was happy that I could immediately answer his questions and show him proof of what he had. It was at this time, I hesitated and asked, "Are you sure? What about [my sister] or [my brother]?" I felt awkward being involved with his finances and wanted to be fair. Despite their lack of involvement, I didn't know what to expect from my sister or brother.

Mardig said he didn't think my sister or brother should be involved. He gave me reasons, which surprised me yet strengthened my willingness to help him.

Days later he would grant me POA over all of his affairs (healthcare and financial).

~:   ~

WE TRIED TO OPEN A BANK ACCOUNT IN CALIFORNIA. Mardig and I went to a neighborhood bank to establish an account in his name. He said since I was his attorney, I should take care of it. I told him he needed to accompany me. We went to the neighborhood bank.

"Hello, I'd like to open up a bank account on behalf of my father."

"Does he have identification?"

"Well, actually no." I'd then lower my voice and add, "He seems to have early Alzheimer's and has misplaced his wallet. However, I do have a POA and I carry identification."

"We cannot open an account for him unless he has identification."

"Well, what do you need?"

"A driver's license or something with a picture ID and his signature."

"He no longer drives."

"Well, *you* could open an account," the customer service representative suggests.

"No, I don't want to do that. I want this to be in his name with me as his POA."

We went through this process with a number of banks. At one point I gave up and started calling banks from home. There was no sense in wasting time visiting each bank. I called instead, "Hello, I've lived here for seven years, shopped at the same neighborhood store, banked at...can you help me?" I was turned down every time.

These rejections started a long and frustrating chase around government bureaucracy and private enterprise. It took one and a half months to get appropriate identification for Mardig.

First, he completed an application at the Social Security office. This required three visits, each entailing a thirty to forty-five minute wait. Next, he completed an application at the Department of Motor Vehicles (DMV) for a California ID. This was accomplished in two visits. Yet we still were uncertain whether he'd receive his ID. We were told his application would be reviewed by a special office in Sacramento. They were uncertain whether his U.S. Citizenship Certificate from the 1930s was an acceptable form of identification because it did not include his birth date. It did, however, note Mardig's age on the date the document was executed. *Simple math would solve this problem. But you can't tell the DMV this!* We decided to apply for a credit card. This would be useful for doctors' visits, clothes shopping, travel, etc. Since Mardig could not open a California bank account, we applied at one of his Milwaukee banks.

Gradually, we acquired items to be included in his wallet.

～   ～

DURING THIS TIME, WE DISCOVERED Mardig's savings bonds had expired. Some of his thirty-plus-year-old savings bonds were no longer earning interest. We made arrangements to cash them to help liquidate funds for his medical care. We couldn't cash them in California—because he still did not have a bank account in the state.

In hindsight, I was glad to have met Mardig's bank representatives in Milwaukee. With a simple phone call, one of these representatives was invaluable in cashing these savings bonds. In California, Mardig would have had to sign each bond in front of a notary of the public. He must have had forty of these bonds. At $5 to $10 per signature, that adds up quickly!

David entered the bonds' serial numbers on the computer, and we sent a copy with the bonds to his Milwaukee bank. Mardig still had to sign each of them. (He was happy to sign them because he kept wanting to cash in all of his accounts to consolidate them into one bank. We didn't think this was a good idea, since he held stock and mutual funds.)

Because the bank in Milwaukee was so helpful, I promised that the proceeds from the cashed bonds would be deposited and left in his account for several months. This was my gesture of appreciation to the bank, since they could make more money off the funds than they paid in interest. Besides, where else could I put the money? We had not yet been able to open a California bank account for Mardig.

Little challenges like these and the constant run-around kept us excessively occupied with his affairs.

A couple months later, the California attorney I retained to advise me on my father's affairs helped me open an account in Mardig's name at a neighborhood bank. *It took five months to open Mardig's first California bank account.*

We also retained a certified public accountant who maintained a ledger and provided an accounting of all my father's finances. Every quarter, we'd gather Mardig's statements and check register and take them to the accountant to copy, so that they could continue updating Mardig's general ledger. This required creating a filing system so that Mardig's records were clearly organized and retrievable. We made it a practice to document everything because we never knew what to expect from my sister and brother.

My aunt and uncle warned me that whenever families deal with money strange things can happen. "People do unreasonable things," they warned. I wanted to keep good records and make certain I was receiving the best advice money could buy. If the need ever arose, I wanted to confidently defend my actions.

∴   ∾

A FEW MONTHS BEFORE MARDIG MOVED TO CALIFORNIA he called to tell me that he thought his car had been stolen. He explained that it had been found, but he had to go claim it. When I asked him if he was going to retrieve it, he said it would cost several hundred dollars to get the car out of the garage. He didn't think it was worth it and decided to forget about it. This didn't make sense to me, because the car was worth several thousand dollars. The best David and I could figure, was that Mardig had driven it somewhere, parked it, forgot about it, and then walked or taken the bus home. We decided the city had it towed to a garage.

I discussed Mardig's lost car with my sister and brother shortly after he mentioned it to David and me. We agreed that it was better for my father not to have a car.

Months later, after Mardig moved in with us, I received a call. His car had been found in a hospital parking lot in a western suburb of Milwaukee. A security guard called and said it had been abandoned. He asked if he could buy it. I told him first I'd like to offer it to my sister. My sister and her husband only had one car, two cars would be a lot more convenient for them.

Even though I communicated infrequently by phone with my sister, I still tried to be considerate. Someday, I thought, she'll respond favorably to my good intentions.

When I called and offered her the car, she was very pleasant and didn't stop talking. This gift, which Mardig granted, inspired a few weeks of conversation and e-mails as we handled the details of transferring the title. She told me it could have been a lot easier had our brother let her into *his* house to look for the title to Mardig's car.

After my sister took ownership of the car, she chastised me for excluding the fair value of the car from her portion of Mardig's annual exclusion gift to her and her husband. *She spat in my face for helping her!* The attorneys had advised me to handle my father's gift in this manner. When I told them of my sister's complaint, they didn't know what to say. *This is a first, attorneys with nothing to say!*

∾   ∾

ANOTHER ONE OF THE LITTLE, YET TIME-CONSUMING, DETAILS THAT remained was learning who really owned Mardig's house. My father frequently shared his fear that my brother owned it and that he had to be careful around him because he didn't want to be left homeless. We weren't sure whose house it was. My brother claimed the house was his. We found undated and unsigned copies of a contract with my brother's name on it. I showed these to the attorney, and he recommended running a title search on the house. We waited for the results. *If the house was my brother's, it would save us a lot of work clearing out so many years' worth of my parents' belongings. We could just leave everything there. If, on the other hand, it was Mardig's, I would have to arrange to clear it out. How long would this take? Who would do this for me? Would they be as meticulous as I would be? When would I find the time? As it is, I have lost business opportunities because of all this work.*

We waited. David and I frequently discussed the pros and cons of the title search report. Meanwhile, we were receiving Mardig's bills since we had filed a "Change of Address" form with the post office. These included utility and property tax bills. If the house belonged to my brother, why was Mardig's name still on these bills? And why were some of the bills marked "overdue?"

We waited and waited, sitting on pins and needles, while we continued processing Mardig's extensive paperwork. *If the house was Mardig's, how would I get my brother to leave after living there his entire life?* David and I hoped my brother owned it. This would be a blessing in disguise.

⌁   ∾

As with most of life's worthy endeavors, our work proved to be challenging. The house was indeed Mardig's. My brother would have to move out so I could sell it. This was not an easy matter—one that simply required my saying, "Dear brother, you've lived in this house for forty-five years for free. Don't you think it's time you moved and went out on your own?"

I had to work out the legalities of evicting a nonrent-paying boarder in Mardig's house. *Yes, there are laws on how to evict a nonpaying boarder!* I sought the advice of Mardig's attorneys and composed a letter to my sister and brother detailing what needed to be done. I invited them to help "dispose" of our parents' personal effects. I was hoping curiosity and the promise of finding treasures in the house would persuade them to get involved. After writing and rewriting the letter a number of times, I finally sent it to both of them with a copy of the POA.

My patience and energy were wearing thin. I was taking care of my father in my home. I was running into problems in every direction. Things were not going as easily as I had expected. And on top of all of this, there were just too many details to take care of!

⌁   ∾

Months passed. My brother eventually moved out. Meanwhile, I took two trips back to Milwaukee to clear out the house and get it ready to sell.

⌁   ∾

BEFORE ARRANGING TO SELL MARDIG'S HOUSE, I asked him, nearly eight months earlier, what he would sell it for if either my sister or brother wanted it. *I thought about buying it, but I lived too far away. It would be a burden to manage from such a distance.*

The house was part of Milwaukee's rich history. It was a two-story, red-brick Colonial built by a banker in 1923. We even found the original blueprints, materials specifications sheets, letters from the original owners, etc., in an old dust-covered box in the corner of the attic. I was impressed to see the care that was given to the selection of materials for the house:

> The mason to furnish and put in the terrazzo finish floors in the front entrance, sunroom, and bathroom, to be of the best grade (guaranteed)...must be put in by thoroughly competent and skilled craftsmen in the art of terrazzo-floor laying. Living, dining room on the first story, and the entire second story...finish floors to be 7/8 x 2 1/4" clean oak...white lead and best linseed oil paint to be used for all painting...front outside door to be solid oak ...front entrance transom to be glazed with zincked glass and a cast not less than $2.00 per foot....

When the appraiser came through the house, he was so taken by it that he described it as a museum piece.

Everything in the house was original. My parents were the second owners and didn't change a thing. The house still had the original boiler, oven and stove, bathtub, sink, and even wallpaper! The inside was generously trimmed in stained solid oak. Even the built-in bookshelves and the majestic mantelpiece were solid oak. The original Edwardian bronze chandelier remained, as did the Edwardian light sconces along the living and dining room walls. Outlining the outside of the house were the original copper drain gutters.

My father said, "Sell it to them between five and ten percent below market value." I had it appraised. Then I had a broker do a detailed market value assessment on it. The broker was generous with her time and the number of comparables she provided.

My sister decided to buy the house, so I gave her a copy of the appraisal. She followed up with a verbal offer, which I accepted because it was within Mardig's requested range. Then she followed up her verbal offer with a written one.

To my surprise, she did what I used to do in the stock market. I'd decide what I wanted to pay for a stock. Then, while I'm actually placing the order, I'd lower the price, hoping that when the stock dipped a little lower it would catch my price. On some occasions, I enjoyed a bigger profit once the stock moved up. Often, however, I missed a generous appreciation using this strategy, and have since placed limit orders closer to the asking price.

My sister's written offer was much lower than her verbal offer. I could not accept her written offer because it was lower than what Mardig wanted. She was not happy when I did not accept her offer. This failed transaction in June marked the end of our future conversations. *I tried communicating with her but she never replied.*

๙   ๛

IN THE COURSE OF LOOKING OVER THE DETAILS, I found a series of checks Mardig had written to an official-sounding organization claiming to preserve Social Security and Medicare. He was sending them checks in response to their official-looking documents. David discovered that over the years, my father's *annual* donations increased to *monthly* and then even *biweekly* payments. We had to put a stop to this. Perhaps it was my naiveté, but I was surprised the organization kept cashing his checks. To our knowledge Mardig's Social Security and Medicare benefits were never threatened.

๙   ๛

WHEN I AGREED TO CARE FOR MY FATHER and signed the POA, I never expected to have so many details to follow up on and process. Initially these tasks took more of David's and my time than Mardig's care.

It is sad that my sister, brother, and I did not communicate easily. I really don't know why. Perhaps it was an issue of trust. I hear stories of how siblings fight bitterly and spitefully, giving away their inheritance to lawyers. Perhaps my sister and brother do not trust me or my handling of our father's affairs. I can understand this. I was told many times that I am the *baby* of the house, and what do I know? I was the first to permanently leave home and move far away. Anticipating their lack of trust, I have kept records of everything and hired specialists to advise me. Someday, long after these issues are resolved, my sister and brother may realize I did everything in the best interest of Mardig and his heirs.

I am confident that my brother and sister would not have had the patience to handle all the details. I don't believe they would have even discovered them in the first place. I recall my brother saying, "I'll just dump everything. I have no time for all this junk. Brenda, I've got a business to run." This *junk* would include my father's U.S. Savings Bonds, information about his accounts around the U.S., and more. All told, this junk would be worth several times what we initially estimated.

Chapter 10

SUPPORT GROUP: WE NEED HELP!

*T*HERE COMES A TIME WHEN EACH OF US MUST FACE our limitations and ask for help. David and I were rapidly approaching that time. It started a few months earlier, when several staff members of the Adult Day Care Center recommended I attend their support group meetings. They suggested this after my repeated requests for advice. "The support group can really help you answer that, Brenda," they'd say each time I asked a question.

I had never been to a *support* group before and felt funny at the thought of sitting around in a circle talking about my problems and listening to everybody else's. I imagined a therapy session or an alcoholics or overeaters anonymous meeting. Besides, I was much too busy. Between trying to manage my father's affairs and trying to grow my soon-to-be non-existent business, where was I to find the time?

⌣ ⌣

A FEW WEEKS LATER, after burning the candle at both ends, I was feeling hopeless. My body was not faring well. I couldn't understand why, with all the care we were giving Mardig, he was declining so quickly. Were we doing something wrong? *Were we not doing enough? What was wrong?*

One day when I dropped him off at the Adult Day Care Center, I raised this question.

Before I left, one of the staff members pulled me aside and painted a vivid picture for me. She said, "Your father is like a drunk who's trying to hold it all together in public. If someone asks him a question, he will answer intelligently. This takes a lot of effort. But once he finally gets in a private place where he feels safe, he loses it. He relaxes and he doesn't always make sense."

It took some time for me to understand her example and to accept analogy. *By doing good for Mardig and making him feel safe and comfortable, we were helping the disease progress. This didn't make sense.*

I still could not focus on building my business. Unable to spend time on my profession, I was increasingly losing patience with Mardig and his affairs. I gave in and went to my first support group meeting the following Tuesday. I *made* the time.

I felt a little awkward at first. I was the youngest attendee among a pool of people in their fifties and older. About half of the participants were caring for their spouses, and the others were caring for their parents. I sat quietly and listened as each shared an update. Then it was my turn to tell my story. The discussion that followed each of our comments proved so invaluable to me I couldn't wait to return. The hour and a half went by much too quickly. I had a page full of ideas.

If your loved one has a hard time getting in and out of the car, place a plastic garbage bag on the seat. This way, he or she can pivot around easily on the slippery bag.

If your loved one is still at home and the bathroom and bedroom doors lock from the inside, make sure to have a small pointed tool handy. I used a tiny jeweler's screwdriver. You can unlock the door from the outside by putting the tool into the tiny hole in the doorknob and jiggling it while twisting the doorknob until it unlocks. This came in handy when Mardig locked himself in the bathroom while taking a shower.

Realize you are now the parent and sometimes you need to be firm with your parent/spouse for his/her own safety.

Get satin sheets for your loved one's bed so he can slide in and out of bed easier. This suggestion was untimely for us. We had just ordered thick flannel sheets so Mardig would be comfortable and warm.

They added, "You will be glad you took on this responsibility in the end." *Yes, if I live that long!*

I attended meetings regularly after this. As my seventeen-year career slowly slipped from my hands, my focus turned toward my father and his care.

The members of the support group became my second family. We shared one important thing in common, one of our family members had Alzheimer's. I believe no one can completely understand what caring for a loved one with Alzheimer's is like without experiencing it. If we used all the words in the world, I doubt we could paint a vivid enough picture of what it is like.

During the days between each support group meeting I jotted questions down about caring for Mardig. Each meeting was so helpful. Each caregiver was at a different stage of the Alzheimer's experience. There was so much we shared. We formed a bond that took us through weeks, and then months, of highs and lows. It is now progressing into years.

Paul, who was in his early eighties, consistently shared at least one profound nugget at each meeting and really made us think.

Patti, who was in her early fifties, cared for her sixty-two-year-old husband. He had the bluest eyes and the most striking wavy white hair I had ever seen.

Jonathan, who, at eighty three, was the oldest person I knew who was progressive enough in his thinking to access the Internet.

I learned later that Paul had also accessed the Internet and was adding features I had not even considered—e.g., voice recognition software and a digital camera.

Paul and Jonathan had each been married to their respective wives for over fifty years before their wives began displaying symptoms of Alzheimer's. Patti enjoyed ten years with Ralph before he began yielding to the clutches of Alzheimer's.

Jeanne, a nurse, gave up her career to care for her mother in her own home. She was in her early fifties.

There were others who attended these meetings, but the participants I've named are the ones who attended consistently and were of the greatest help to me.

It is often said, when talking about families and the family members' loyalty to each other, that "blood is thicker than water." Unfortunately, this has not been my experience. I harbor the pain of not having a supportive relationship with my sister and brother. I would like to argue that if blood is thicker than water, so what? *Water is the fluid of life!*

The support group and the book, *The 36-Hour Day*, written by Nancy L. Mace and Peter V. Rabins, were two key items in my caregiver survival kit. *The 36-Hour Day* could be easily called the caregiver's Bible. The cover on my copy reads, "A family guide to caring for persons with Alzheimer's disease, related dementing illness, and memory loss in later life." Each of us who wanted to survive had our own copies, which we would refer to each time something new happened that we could not understand. Sometimes the answers weren't specific enough. Other times, they were painfully graphic.

During a particularly trying week in October 1996 I wanted to ask the question everyone asks at some time, "When will I know I can't do it alone anymore?"

To try and make sense of it at a later date, I wrote the details of this difficult week in my journal.

October 1996

Last night was awful...I was very sick. The flu hit me severely, and Mardig was not being cooperative. He went to bed around 10:00 p.m. and so did I. I was having terrible chills. The quartz heater was tuned on "high" to warm me under three covers and I still could not combat the chills. David was cleaning up the kitchen after he made chicken soup for us.

David came to bed about 10:30. Mardig was in his room and the lights were turned off. At 11:00, we noticed the lights go on. Hell was about to begin...

He got out of his room, all dressed, and was ready to leave. He started wandering around in the house wearing his shoes.

He was opening doors, cupboards, including the front door eight times (it makes a squeaky noise so we knew). I didn't want to get up because I was freezing. Mardig quietly went into the utility room and turned on the lights and then turned them off. We couldn't make sense of what we were *not* hearing. He must have just stood there in the dark. David got up and peered down the hallway from our bedroom door. Who knows what my father was doing. I feared that he might hurt himself. (I think we need to childproof this house so he doesn't get hurt.)

After that, David got up six or seven times. It was 3:00 a.m. and David had to get up in an hour to leave by 4:55 a.m. He was too exhausted. He just couldn't take it anymore. I got up at 3:30 a.m. and looked around.

David's files of his parents' tax and business records had been opened. The organized piles on my desk had been mixed up. Each pile was for a different project. It took me time to organize my work. During the few hours I had each day to work, I certainly didn't have time to reorganize after someone else messed my files! I was cold, very cold. I lost patience. What happens if I get hurt or truly can't get up? How will I take care of my father? This was inappropriate...Mardig was causing too much trouble. Battling severe chills, I had enough...I confronted Mardig and told him this couldn't go on any longer. He told me to leave him alone. I said I couldn't because he was messing up my stuff and affecting my life! He told me to leave him be that he would die soon. *Oooohhh, the ultimate in guilt-rendering tactics had been employed!*

The following morning, I found a little block of bittersweet baking chocolate on the floor by the kitchen sink. (We keep it in the cupboards high above Mardig's head.) I found a spoon in the toaster. (It's a good thing we are in the habit of unplugging the toaster.) When I told Mardig about this he was amazed and denied he'd do anything so stupid—"You could get a shock!" he added. I found the jar of peanut butter among the cleaning supplies under the sink.

Later that day, he pulled out another slice of bread from the bag, after I had already given him a slice to have with his soda. (He liked to eat bread and wash it down with sweet creamy soda.) When I came into the kitchen, both pieces of bread were placed on the cats' feeding dish, which was at the edge of the counter. I made him aware of what he had done. He thanked me for looking out for him. I threw the bread out for the birds and retrieved another couple of slices for him. *I have to constantly keep an eye on him so he doesn't harm himself.*

We will have to try sleeping pills for Mardig. We'll see how they help him sleep. It'll be good for him and us. This was recommended by other caregivers at the support group meeting. As it would turn out, the sleeping pills worked the first night he took them. The second and third nights he was up wandering, so we stopped giving him sleeping pills after the third night.

I have decided to start researching our options for assisted care for him. We'll check one out this weekend. It is just too difficult constantly watching him each time he gets up.

I feel the dual emotions of sadness and relief...David says Mardig is 86. He's lived his life, now we must live ours. I agree. On the other hand, he seems so helpless, so innocent. His being here has taught me so much about options. Life is full of them! And it's not like he's doing this on purpose. Yeah, sometimes he's ornery just to be stubborn, but most of the time he doesn't realize he's being bothersome.

So, it was after these incidents that I first brought the question to my support group family. "How do you know when you can't do it anymore? When you just can't care for your loved one."

"You'll know," one said. "We can't tell you, because it's different for everyone," Paul added.

I was disappointed with his reply. *What an easy way to get off with-*

out answering the question in a genuinely helpful manner. That's not what I needed, especially from my second family! I had never done this before. How will I know when I can't do it anymore?

✻ ✻

OVER THE MONTHS, I WAS TO LEARN HOW RIGHT THEY WERE. Each of us knows our limits. There were many times during the five months my father lived with us that we wanted to give up. "Let's just take him back to Milwaukee and leave him there," we'd say after a particularly difficult day. "We don't owe him anything! We've already given him more than anyone else in the family has."

We couldn't take him back. We had taken on a responsibility. We had to see it through. David and I made many sacrifices. Weekends and evenings devoted to my father's care. It wasn't having a positive impact on our relationship either.

All of this was exhausting...Mardig's erratic sleep schedule, increased disorientation and confusion, and bouts of incontinence. David went to work each day, while I stayed at home, being a parent to my sick father who had caught the flu.

Mardig had refused to stay away from me while I was sick. He'd touch my hand and then eat without washing his hands. "What's a little germ?" he'd reply, when David and I would urge him to wash his hands.

Mardig experienced two significant rounds of incontinence; once, when he caught the flu and the second time, after he ate dry cat food. When he had the flu we were concerned about keeping his fever down. I called the doctor in a panic when his fever rose up to 103° with no signs of abating. The doctor advised using Tylenol®. It worked quickly. Every few hours when his temperature started creeping back up I'd take his temperature and give him Tylenol®. He was very confused as to when and how to use the bathroom. He was uncertain of the time of day. He was not communicating clearly.

And so I was to discover the depths of my compassion and caring for my father. Fecal matter fell out of his pant leg as he walked with me to the bathroom. I helped him to the toilet and then went back to clean up the mess. I stepped on some in his bedroom. *Yuck! Human feces!*

He ate the dry cat food we kept on the counter in a sealed plastic container. *So much for the elderly being so poor they eat dog food. My father's eating cat food!* He became so constipated he had a bowel movement whenever he could. We found fecal bits in his bedroom, in the hallway, and some twenty steps away in the living room. *We definitely needed to have the carpets cleaned.*

◡ ◡

I WOULD WAKE AT 4:30 EACH MORNING with the goal of getting some work done. First, I'd check his bathroom. "It was easier to clean a small mess than a big one," I reasoned. I found feces and urine on the floor and his soiled underwear in the sink. *If his underwear was in the sink, what was he (not) wearing?* I began each morning with a bottle of bleach, plenty of paper towels, and wiped his bathroom clean. What a way to start each day.

We knew the time was coming soon when we could not keep him in our home any longer.

◡ ◡

THROUGH ALL THESE HIGHS AND LOWS, the support group became invaluable to me. Without my second family I would have felt alone, misunderstood, and in foreign territory. Frankly, I would not have been able to get through it. These were people who candidly shared their experiences and helped me understand what Mardig was going through. By sharing their knowledge they helped me anticipate what to expect from my father. They had already tried everything. By sharing their experiences they helped me care for Mardig more easily. In turn, I too provided them ideas, as I learned. *It isn't very hard to develop knowledge in this area over a brief period of time. In just a few intense months, I had gained enough experience to give advice to newcomers.*

John Bradshaw said, "When you become a member of a support group, stay with it at least a year and up to three to get the full benefit out of it." I agree. One or two meetings won't help. You're developing a trusting relationship with others about very personal issues. It takes time to grow a mutual respect and trust, and the emotional bonds that accompany such meaningful relationships. So, I did. I started one meeting at a time and developed a relationship with people who had been meeting months, perhaps years, before I joined their family.

I'm glad I did…for my father's sake and mine!

PART III

Drowning In Uncertainty

Chapter 11

THE MOST DIFFICULT DECISION

In January 1997, fraught with uncertainty about the future, David and I faced the most difficult decision yet about my father's care. We gave more detailed consideration to this decision than we did months earlier when we moved my father into our home.

$\mathcal{D}$AVID AND I LAID OUT ALL OUR OPTIONS FOR MY FATHER'S CARE. We then evaluated the appropriateness and the probability of success of each. We were left with three choices:

1. Buy a bigger house. My uncle suggested David and I use what was left of my father's assets to buy a nice comfortable home for the three of us. When Mardig first moved to California, he talked about buying a place of his own. If we bought a larger home with his assets, we realized we'd be living off of him. We did not feel comfortable doing this. We also felt that my brother and sister would complain if they knew we were benefiting financially. Besides, we didn't want to be stuck with the added responsibility of selling the house to settle the estate after Mardig died.

   One of the members in the support group had done this. Her mother purchased a large house. She and her family (husband and children) live upstairs and her mother lives downstairs. Over time, her mother became verbally abusive toward her. Her mother's outbursts were painful and disturbing for the family.

Yet, because she was living in her mother's house, she felt trapped with the obligation to care for her mother.

A justification for buying a larger home was that we could hire a full-time live-in caregiver for Mardig. We'd need someone at least sixteen hours per day. One person could not work this many hours. An alternative could be to hire several caregivers to work in shifts. But then we'd have to take time to find qualified people. *How would we be able to determine the extent of someone's qualifications for such a job?* It would be a process of trial and error. *Who had this kind of time?* Then we'd have to deal with all of the employment issues—e.g., workers' compensation, taxes, etc. If we went through an agency, the costs would be higher, and we still wouldn't be sure of the quality or dependability. What if David and I were out of town on business and the person didn't show up for his/her shift?

A related option is that *we* could buy a larger home. We didn't want to move into a larger house. Given the fickleness of the real estate market in our area, we did not want to allocate our personal funds toward such an investment.

2. Place Mardig in a board and care home. The homes we had visited consisted of a couple who lived in a large house and cared for a handful of residents who lived with them. This would also be a personal approach. We could even visit my father. *But what about the occasional abuses we had heard about—or the neglect?* We could monitor this by making unannounced visits. *But how could we really be sure?* Still, this looked like an attractive option—a warm and comfortable home with a family atmosphere.

   All we needed to do was find a good family. This was easier than we thought, because we found one right in our neighborhood. The family seemed kind. The only hindrance was that they took care of incapacitated, elderly females. My father was neither. Also, the brick wall surrounding their house was only four-feet tall. Mardig wandered and could easily get over this wall. We continued looking for a board and care home where the owners locked their doors so that wanderers like my father could not get out. During our search we learned that locking doors to prevent residents from walking out required special state licensing because of emergency exit requirements. The homes we visited were not licensed by the state.

3. Consider a skilled nursing facility. Months earlier we had driven around the perimeter of a nearby facility and were upset by the prospect of people living in an institutional environment. Weeks later, Mardig, David, and I took a tour of the facility. It was *very* institutional—white walls, sterile environment, and the overwhelming smell of cleaning solution. It was certainly clean. When we asked about the strong smell, we were told the residents became disoriented and occasionally urinated in the hallways or in their rooms. The facility combated this behavior by constantly cleaning.

How could we pull my father out of our nice warm home, with plush carpeting, soft recliners, a warm bed with flannel sheets and a down comforter—to throw him into such a sterile facility with cold tile floors and white walls? It was painful to even consider this. When we completed the tour, Mardig asked, "Was that for me?"

"Yes," we answered honestly, amazed at his candor and fearful he would react negatively.

"It'll be a good place to live once I retire," he added. Hearing this gave us some comfort.

After all, we justified, he would have twenty-four-hour care in a state-licensed facility. This should ensure plenty of supervision and that there would be no abuse.

↲　↳

WEEKS LATER, WE DECIDED THE THIRD OPTION WOULD BE THE BEST and safest.

Less than a week before Mardig was admitted, David and I struggled with the choice we had made. We had a business trip planned in February, and Mardig would need to be looked after. The experimental drug was not improving his ability as we had hoped. We drew partial comfort from the realization that if Mardig's condition improved, we could have him return to our home. We arranged to admit Mardig one week before we left on our trip, to make sure things worked out all right. If they didn't, we'd have to find another solution. If his condition improved, we would bring him home. This thought helped us deal with the pain of having to leave Mardig. The greatest difficulty was in how we would break the news to him. *He would not be sleeping in his warm soft bed. He would no longer share breakfasts and dinners with us. Would he survive? How would he react?*

The stress and inner turmoil was killing me. Once again, I began writing my thoughts in my journal.

January 24, 1997

A day of emotional highs and lows...a lot of emotional stretch...

Last night, we heard the hum of Mardig's battery powered wet-dry razor. This meant he was getting ready to go to *work*. David told him we were going to bed because it was night time. Mardig laughed it off as he does when he doesn't agree. He must have stayed up for quite a bit!

Walked in Mardig's bedroom at 7:45 a.m. He was sleeping. This was unusual...but then again he thought it was morning last night. I asked him to get up. He wanted to sleep for 10 more minutes. I told him I had a 9:00 a.m. appointment and that it was 8:32 and if he slept for 10 minutes I would surely be late. He said, "Okay," and I extended my hand to help him get up. He got up without my assistance and said my fingers were too thin and that he would fall if he were to grab my hand. *Hmmm.*

He got ready quickly and immediately asked for his shoes. (This question had grated on us for a while now.)

We left for the VNA Adult Day Care Center. I dropped him

off at the door and Ellie, who was standing outside, took him in.

At 9:00 a.m. I went to the attorney's office to discuss matters pertaining to Mardig's estate—getting the items in his house appraised, appraisers, gifts, etc. I had carefully sorted my notes and created a list of items in priority order. At $200 an hour, I needed to get in and out of there, quick!!!

At 10:15 a.m. I went to the skilled nursing facility to complete a mound of admittance forms for my father. It was shortly before noon when we completed nearly an inch of paperwork. The admissions representative was kind enough to mail the forms to us in advance, and David and I read each page and wrote questions/comments in the margins. This way I could address specific issues when I came into her office. I was trying to be efficient. The representative said other family members did not ask so many questions nor notice such detail. (I have Mardig's genes). Still, the reality of this preparation was too much for me to bear. I was able to concentrate on the paperwork and repress what was happening to my body while in her office. Before leaving, I had the opportunity to meet Mardig's future doctor and talk with him for a few minutes.

When I completed the paperwork and left the facility, my body began to shake. I lost my sense of orientation. I couldn't think. It was after the noon hour and I needed to go west to the office supply store to buy paper. I froze. I didn't know where to go next. I never thought to look in my calendar to see what was next on my list. Those who know me know that looking in my calendar is as natural for me as breathing. I called home and checked for messages. There were none. So I headed south to the credit union to take care of some long overdue finances—transferred some funds, and withdrew some cash.

On the way home I felt a sense of relief that I had taken care of Mardig's affairs with the attorney and the skilled nursing facility.

I knew in my heart I was doing everything I possibly could for him. I knew someday everything would be scrutinized because of the precarious relationship between my siblings and me. I've always maintained that I will do the best I know how based on the expert advice I receive so that I can stand up and defend my actions.

Yet, the future holds unexpected surprises and uncertainties...

Monday, January 27, 1997   5:29 a.m.

I could not sleep any longer. David left at 4:29 this morning in order to put in more hours so we could go together when Mardig was admitted to the skilled nursing facility on Thursday. Thoughts raced through my mind about *the* day when we would have Mardig admitted.

Last night David and I had a long discussion about our feelings and thoughts of telling Mardig in advance. *It is our moral obligation and the right thing to do...not to mention, we'd feel better about being up front and truthful. On the other hand, Mardig won't remember the details, but may remember the feeling associated with hearing such news. He may ask the same questions repeatedly and even feel upset.* If we do tell him, what do we say? If my brother were here right now, he'd say, "Hey, Mardig, you're going into a nursing home." If we told him the truth, we'd say, "We are going to have you stay there awhile under the doctor's observation and with people who will help you be more active. Since you are on the experimental drug study, this may increase your chances for improvement. Additionally, David and I will be on travel and away from home for two weeks, and we want to make sure you are being cared for—that your meals are prepared and that you have your other needs taken care of."

The uncertainty of how he will respond was distracting us and keeping us awake. *This is a free country and even a person with Alzheimer's who has granted his daughter with POA over his affairs and healthcare has the right to refuse admission into a nursing facility.*

So what do we do?

Anyway, this morning I lay awake, my mind swirling with thoughts, "What other items did I need to add to Mardig's resident contract to make sure all his needs are documented and looked after? I need to reread and write notes on his six-page resident rights document." I was also thinking about what to take with us (e.g., clothes, personal effects) when he gets admitted Thursday. I was thinking about which friends I could call who would visit him while we were away.

Sigh. This is all for now. Time to make some coffee. (5:40 a.m.)

I started videotaping the days before we were to admit Mardig into the skilled nursing facility. On January 26, 1997, we were waiting for Dave and Jan to arrive to watch the Green Bay Packers win their third Super Bowl. It would be four to one with all of us former Wisconsinites (Jan, Mardig, David and me) against the former Pennsylvanian, Dave. Mardig was sitting at the dining room table reading the Sunday paper while trying to shoo away Djermag, our white cat, who shares his affinity for newspapers. Mardig likes to read them. Djermag likes to roll around on them.

I wanted to capture as many moments as I could with my father. The next time I'd videotape him would be the evening before he was to go to the skilled nursing facility. I had struggled for three days and couldn't bring myself to tell him where he was going. Yet, I had to. I owed it to him.

Wednesday, January 29, 1997

I woke up early and started working at 4:50. Lots on my mind, stomach in knots, acid, burning. Took Rolaids. From the separation anxiety of losing a family member, to other issues with people whose behavior and decisions I was trying to understand.

Mardig and I greeted each other at about 5:00 a.m. after I heard his hearing aid whistling. The high-pitched tone had awakened David and me many times during the past months. Mardig would take his hearing aid out and leave it turned on. If something was placed near it, the feedback would cause it to whistle. When I went in his room to turn it off, I noticed he was up. I encouraged him to go back to bed. To my surprise, he said, "For you, I will." I thought, "Why do you have to be so sweet and cooperative the day before you're to leave us?" I helped tuck him under the covers.

I went into my office to start working.

Shortly, he got up to go to the bathroom. He came into my room and asked the formidable question that wreaks terror in David's and my hearts, "Where's my shoes?"

Once again, I encouraged him to go back to bed after we talked briefly. He declined, saying he'd rather stay up since he'd already been to bed several times before. He went to the living room and sat on the recliner.

I resumed my work. I had looked for e-mail from my sister last night and this morning. None. I had sent her an e-mail explaining the situation—we were going on business travel and Mardig needed to be watched. I wished she would have written something. Nothing. *Gotta go this journey alone.*

David and I talked about my brother. To our amazement he had not called at all. David asked if I will call or contact him. I suppose I should. One of us has to try to behave maturely. Besides, every family has a member like him—lives free of rent and utilities, never calls or writes to see how his father is, received a sizable sum of cash via questionable means, claims closeness to his mother while reaping benefits and then never shows up when she dies. But then again, neither did my sister. *How do families get like this? I thought we grew up close.* If anyone should have turned her back, it should have been me! I left at 18, never received any help, and never moved back.

I got up to make myself some hot chocolate. I figure I'll drink it to soothe my upset stomach and to warm up. Been having the chills for the last 12 hours! Must be the stress given what we're about to do to my father. Then I realize Mardig must also feel like me. I should make him some. This is his second last morning here. This sends tremors through me. "It's not like he's going to die! It's not like I'll never see him again," I keep repeating to myself. Still, it's a major change for him and us. So, I'll bring him some warm chocolate milk with honey. He loves sweet things.

Shall I stay and talk with him? Spend together time? Or shall I continue writing my thoughts here? I know once he's been away awhile that I will have more time, patience, and energy for him. Yet, when one requires so much of your attention and thoughts, his sudden absence will create a major void because your efforts are no longer required.

Time to get his cocoa and talk with him a bit.   (6:47 a.m.)

That evening, after torturing myself as to how I would tell Mardig he would be living someplace else temporarily, I told him I wanted to vidcotape him. It was important to me to capture this emotionally difficult and life-changing moment on tape. He said, "Okay."

I was nervous. I didn't know how to begin. He asked what I wanted him to do. I invited him to have a seat. Once I had the camera set up and he and I were settled, I began by asking him general questions about his day.

"What did you do today?"

"I was trying to read the *People's*...uh, *People's* manual..."

"...the *People's Almanac*," I filled in.

"Yeah."

"So what did you do today?" I asked again. "Do you remember?"

"Really, I didn't do anything. You did everything."

"So what did you do?" I repeated emphasizing *you*.

"Well, you took me to the doctor. We got the doctor to say that I'm not falling apart." (He went to the podiatrist.)

"We went to the new place," he continued.

I didn't know what he was referring to, so I asked him another question. "Do you remember what you did...at the building behind the church?" This is what we called the Adult Day Care Center.

"Yeah."

"Did they throw you a party?" Roberta said they would have a little party for him since it was his last day. I assumed they had, so I tried to jar his memory.

"Nah!" he said chuckling. "They wouldn't throw anyone a party. If I were graduating, I would have to come in the door and throw them a party. On the other hand if I'm just leaving, 'Good riddance. We gotta make room for someone else,'" he said pretending they were talking.

Our generic discussion continued. Painfully, I tried to be patient, yet wanted ever so much to talk with him about what was to happen to him. I was trying to find a way to smoothly transition into telling him. When I just couldn't, and felt tormented enough, I went ahead and started.

"Mardig, doesn't it interest you that it's your last day...do you wonder why?" I asked awkwardly.

He started coughing and said, "When you say 'your last day,' keep in mind what you mean..." He got up to spit. He returned and continued, "When you say, 'last day'...I don't get what you mean 'last day.'"

I didn't know what to say. I felt so uncomfortable. "Well, you know how you've been going to the center every day. Every day you've been going to the center..."

"Yeah..."

"And today is your last day."

"How's that?"

"Because tomorrow you're going to start another thing," I was being evasive. I didn't know how to say what needed to be said.

"The what?" he asked. Even with his hearing aid, he constantly questioned what he thought he heard.

I repeated, "Because tomorrow you're going to start something else."

"Oh, that's interesting. Tell me about it," he said. "I may not like it, but tell me." *This last comment didn't make it any easier.*

"Well, I hope you like it," I tried to be as enthusiastic as possible. "Uh, tomorrow you're going to be going to the...hold on a moment, I want to do something." I had to make sure there was enough tape left in the camera. *What an awkward time to have to stop. It was hard enough getting this far!*

He began humming as he watched me. He hummed when he was happy or nervous. Then he broke the awkward silence, "A little while ago when you said that...ahhhh...as close as we are...sometimes, I don't...hey, she's a girl!" He looked at David who had just joined us.

"Yeah! Yeah!" I said agreeing with him that I am a girl. *He had been having difficulty recognizing my gender. He routinely commented on how cute I was and that I would have no trouble finding a partner. He even tried to match me up with female staff members and volunteers at the Adult Day Care Center.*

"That never occurs to me, there's a difference there. Let's keep the difference..."

I humored him. "She has girl parts and you have boy parts," I said.

"That ought to make it even, huh?" he joked.

I was trying desperately to tell him about how his life was going to be different starting tomorrow. I continued, "So tomorrow you begin another phase of your life. Tomorrow we will take you to a place where they will observe you...there will be doctors who will observe you." *All the advice we received suggested using this strategy to tell Mardig that he was going someplace. They advised that we should play it one day at a time. Tell him he'll be there for one or two days. While he's there, the staff will stretch out the time to three and four days and then one week, one month, etc. I felt so sad. I was betraying him. There he sat so trusting, so innocent, so helpless!*

I mustered the courage to continue. "Remember when we put you on that experimental drug study?"

"Are we done with that?"

"No, that'll keep going on for a while."

"The little white, the...well we still have that. I got some today, even," he said.

"No, yesterday, last night you got some," I clarified needlessly. I felt so uncomfortable and tried hard not to show it.

"Well, it's a continuation of that, in other words, it's the same level of whacha m'call..." he volunteered. He was making this easier on me. *Why should he? I was betraying him!*

"Well, this is a place where you will stay in residence, which means you'll spend the night there."

"Oh!"

"It will go across several days."

"Oh!"

"And you'll be part of daily activities. There's a large staff there, and they will take you through daily activities. The hope is that keeping you stimulated and continuing this experimental drug study that perhaps there might be some improvement." *My brain was working like a wet noodle. Yet, if I stopped talking I knew I would fall apart. I kept the momentum going. I had to get it out. He had to hear what I needed to say. I felt I was betraying him and if I could keep talking maybe somewhere in my words there would be something that he'd like. I continued.* "The reason why we're doing this at this time is because David and I will be leaving town for a little bit."

"Oh really, how long will you be gone?"

"Two weeks," I emphasized, "and we're going to have to make arrangements for someone to look after you while we are away." *How could I have said this?*

"Child of the house, you mean," he said with a nervous chuckle.

His hand covered his mouth. During the entire conversation, except when he gestured, he covered his mouth with his left hand. This was unusual for him. He usually let his arms and hands rest on the armrests of the rocking chair.

"Well, not really, but because you're disoriented we need to help you."

"No, don't...don't...I understand," he tried to let me off the hook.

"Are you aware of it?" I wanted to know if he knew he was disoriented.

"No, I don't know what you said, but there's a difference when you…ahh…reach a certain stage…first you're a kid. I treat you as a kid, you're nobody. I mean, I can be impersonal with you and you're supposed to take all that and then suddenly you don't talk with her…"

"Well, you haven't said anything inappropriate," I volunteered. When he saw me as a man, he would comment on the appearance of women, and then play matchmaker.

"Well, I…"

"You're a diplomat," I added. "You were one when I was a little girl and you continue to be one." I wanted to compliment him. "I just wanted you to be aware. You'll stay at this place and they will evaluate your progress. In February there will be a specialist who will come from Granada Hills to evaluate you. When she…"

"She?"

"Yes, she'll be coming up. When she comes up, David and I will be out of town, so you have to behave," I said humorously.

"Well, it's hard to say if I disbehave(sic)! Well," he chuckled mischievously, "I'll be acting like any other *he* person," he said, emphasizing his male gender.

"All men are alike, right?" I was feeling less anxious.

"Right," he agreed.

"I just wanted you to know because it will change your life for a bit. You've been spending nights with us, but because they will be observing you, you will not be spending nights with us."

"Oh, where will I be?"

"You'll be just four miles from our house."

"Oh," he said, his hand still covering his mouth.

"Can I walk that?"

"No, we'll come."

"Well, I can handle that, especially when it's not raining."

This was all I wanted to discuss about the following day with him. I switched subjects and tried to get him to answer some simple questions regarding his awareness. This would be a good benchmark before the disease progressed further.

"Do you know what state we're in?"

"Now, we're going to get into trouble," he chuckled and looked at David. We had discussed this so many times during the past weeks. He just couldn't believe he was in California.

"Well, what state are we in?" I repeated.

"Geography says," he chuckled, "name."

"What side of the country are we in?" I tried to make it easier on him.

"On the east side of the country," he replied.

"In what state?"

"New York."

"We're on the east side of the country in New York?" I inquired for clarification.

"Quite a bit of New York is in this part of the country...well the fact that I have a bank there that's still on the water and it hasn't moved...last I heard I still have the same name."

I thought I'd switch the topic to his family. "How many children do you have?"

"Oh, this gets to be big," he replied looking at David and then back at me.

"No, how many children do you have?"

"Three of them," he said confidently.

"What are their names?"

"[My brother's name]...ahhh, what is the duke's name?"

I didn't know to whom he was referring. "How many boys? How many girls?"

"Three boys and one girl," he said quickly.

"That's four," I said. "Earlier you said you had three kids."

He hesitated.

"How many children do you have?" I thought I'd try again.

"You're one..." and then he added, "Brenda. There's one a little further north of us and there's another one that I've got a very casual relationship with him...I don't think I've even seen his face."

"What are your kids' names?"

"Brenda," he said.

"What's the middle child's name?"

"Uhhhh."

"Your daughter…you have two daughters and one son."

"And one son?" he asked. "Hey, what did you do with the other son?" he smiled.

"You've never had another son. At least, let me put it this way, in all the years I've lived in that house I never knew of another son of yours. Now, if you have another son on the side, I'll turn off the video-camera and we can talk about it."

We giggled.

"Is that a video?"

"Yeah, we can watch it on TV later…you can see yourself on TV, later." I had to repeat things frequently and keep my comments brief since he had trouble hearing.

"Really look foolish, huh?" he said.

"Nahhh, why did you say that?" I inquired. *I was just starting to feel less awful about what we were about to do to him and then he says this.*

"Sarcastic," was his one-word answer.

"Oh."

"Disgruntled and unable to man yourself," he added.

Our black cat, the one who likes to cuddle, came into the room. I picked her up and placed her on his lap. A pleasant distraction, I hoped. He didn't want her to sit on his lap, "I don't want that stranger here." He always feared our *girls* (our three cats) would relieve them-selves on him.

"Who's idea is this, all yours?" he asked out of the clear blue.

"What?" *I didn't understand.*

"To straighten me out."

How do I answer such a direct question? "I'm trying to see what can happen for you because I think you might enjoy…"

"Well, I may have some female tactics in me."

This took me by surprise. "Explain," I said.

"Childish, let's say."

"You do? Inside of you?" I inquired.

"Yeah, well because my freedom has generally been with females and since you were also part of the family and very close and also a female, the fact that you were female was completely erased off of you and …you male."

"Well, I'm trying to find ways to help you improve if that's possible…" I said, not understanding the point he was trying to make.

"I don't object," he interrupted.

"…it would be good if you can. You see, the disease of Alzheimer's is a disintegrating disease. But…there are drugs or certain therapies that can help you improve a little bit. There are places that have more activities than we can provide. You come here and read but you don't get enough stimulation, walking around and…" *I was making as little sense as he was!*

Our black cat came in again and jumped on his bed. I drew his attention to her.

"Get off of there," he demanded. She ignored him.

"Ohhhh, look at the kitty cat," I teased.

"Get off of there," he repeated.

"Nahhh," I teased some more. "Look at her curl up so comfy on your soft fluffy covers."

Our white cat came in and headed for his closet. The *girls* had distracted us. I stopped the videocamera.

I felt better than I would have had I not said anything at all. Still, I felt uncomfortable with the situation. I knew in my heart I was misrepresenting the situation to my father. Sure, I was told, it was for his own good. Nevertheless, I knew what I was doing and it didn't feel right.

That night David and I did not sleep. Mardig, on the other hand, slept soundly. We didn't hear him get up. I wanted to videotape everything the following morning, but I was so tired and nervous about what we were going to do that I didn't want anything to mess up an already difficult situation. I did, however, manage to videotape a brief portion of David shaving Mardig. He dressed himself, but had not shaved, so David carefully shaved his face as I made stupid comments,

trying to detract from our feelings of awkwardness. The tape will provide us with a warm and touching video of a son-in-law and his father-
in-law.

Thursday, January 30, 1997   4:25 p.m.

Well, we did it...we took Mardig to the skilled nursing facility.
We arrived at 9:00 a.m., exactly one-half hour after our
appointment. He walked in willingly following us a few paces
behind as he frequently did during the past few months. The
social services representative pleasantly greeted him with a big
smile and asked if he would come with her. He walked with
her through the double doors.

We watched as he crossed the threshold, *the threshold*...the
locked doors from which he cannot get out unless someone
signs him out and escorts him. Wow, what a transition in our
lives—*his* and ours!

It was difficult and I had paid my dues. I had agonized over
this for the past two days—didn't eat, couldn't sleep, was upset
emotionally, and even had diarrhea. David wasn't feeling all
that good either! But now that Mardig was admitted, I began
feeling better.

It was a *passing* of sorts. He passed from one place in his life
to another. My feelings were even stronger about this passing
than the uncertain transition of his life from Milwaukee to
California.

Now he is in the skilled nursing facility and he thinks he's
there under observation for a day or two. The social services
director, who was quite pleasant and charming, assured us
that this was okay, and the staff will gradually stretch out this
observation period. This seemed so deceiving. Yet, for the person with Alzheimer's, this is all they know. It is sad. The ultimate betrayal.

Jonathan and Patti were there to visit their spouses and to
show us support. I told the support group earlier that we would
be admitting my father on this day. Jonathan had just endured

the pain of admitting his wife, Elizabeth, a few weeks earlier. He knew exactly what we were experiencing. Jonathan waved to us from the other side of the door when we arrived. Once we saw him, he offered to take us out to lunch after we admitted Mardig. We accepted. He helped us deal with this difficult transition.

Patti told us later she tried to greet us while we were in a closed-door meeting with the social services director. Patti's husband, Ralph, looks so endearingly at her. Actually, today is the second time I saw him. The special way he looks at Patti is permanently etched in my mind—head tilted, baby blue eyes lovingly open, and a slight smile. It's a look of, "How sweet it is to see you, my love." I am sure he was a heartthrob. It must have been very hard for her to have him admitted two years ago.

The admission process was thorough. The process lasted from 9:00 a.m. to 12:45 p.m. I found that being detailed, something I inherited from my father, was useful—detailed notes, plenty of questions, etc. In a way, I honored Mardig by asking questions and taking notes. He took detailed notes during my childhood. Now, I'm doing the same for him. Furthermore, I am requesting all records kept on him—psycho-social assessment, admission history, etc.

The psycho-social assessment with the social services director consisted of questions about Mardig one year prior to admission to the facility and about his lifestyle during his earlier years. "Reads everything, likes to do things with his hands—mechanical, electrical, functional things," she wrote on the form. "He didn't do as much with the family since he worked a lot." The social services director asked if he had other children.

"Two more," I said.

She asked if they would visit.

"It's unlikely," I said with some degree of confidence. *It is sad, but after writing to my sister that we were going to admit him, we have heard nothing, not even an acknowledgment that she received the message. During this time, the attorney sent my father's annual exclusion gift to her. Perhaps we may hear from her soon?*

We inquired why these questions were being asked. The social services director told us that this information helps to establish a benchmark for Mardig's condition upon admission and that it stays on record in the event of a lawsuit.

"A lawsuit?" David asked.

"Yes," she said, and explained that family members may insist that they've visited everyday and played an active part in the person's life when, for example, trying to negotiate an estate settlement.

We also met with the nursing supervisor. We had to make a decision regarding Mardig's healthcare needs. Do we want him to be revived, sustained, etc.? We opted to customize the simple form. Instead of saying a generic "yes" or "no," we opted for CPR in the facility and then, once he was taken to the hospital and we received the doctor's diagnosis, we would determine the degree of life-sustaining measures necessary. *When I think about it, the ramifications of a simple "yes" or "no" are amazing! What if his heart stopped for a minor reason and we said "No" on the form? He would not be revived and left to die. If we don't give him this option, he has no chance, period.*

Mardig had prepared us. He shared his opinions regarding life-saving measures. I remember these discussions well. They occurred in the kitchen and in the basement of his Milwaukee home. He'd say he didn't want his life prolonged if the situation was irreversible and terminal. Regardless of what we feel, we believe that this is *his* life and *his* decision on how he wants to live it and when he wants to die. We will determine whether he should have an IV, a feeding tube, etc., once his doctor makes the diagnosis in the hospital. In essence, he would say, "If the prognosis is terminal and life-support is the only way I can survive, let me die."

Sally just made this decision about her father. In answer to his wish, she asked that he not be put on dialysis. His kidneys were weak and not functioning. He would live until toxins (filtered by healthy kidneys) overwhelmed his body, and then he would die. She struggled with this, because she felt she had sentenced the last member of her forebears to death. When the time comes, I hope to have her strength.

I occasionally wonder if my sister and brother could make these decisions. I assumed they would not give Mardig's wishes as much consideration as I had. This assumption gave me strength as I played the role of my father's lone legal advocate. I remember my brother telling the hospital not to let anyone else see or talk with my mother (not even my sister and me) when her prognosis went downhill. He pushed us away when our family needed to be together. My sister, on the other hand, breaks down and cries. She gets too emotional in my opinion and doesn't exercise good judgment. When I claim she's taking the easy route with all her displays of helpless emotion, people tell me to be more understanding of her. I can't. I mean who says I am so strong? Again, I try to convince myself that this is just life. What we get out of life is what we put into it. *Right now, I'm putting in too much!*

It's 5:43 p.m. and David is pressure cooking some lima beans, for our southern style dinner with Lew this evening. I hear the "shhhhhhh" sound from the steam escaping. I wonder, "What's Mardig doing now?" I want to run into his room and see, but he's no longer there.

Chapter 12

THE GREAT ESCAPE!

I included this chapter with some degree of trepidation because my father still resides at the facility where "The Great Escape" occurred. However, initial reviewers of this book urged me to include this chapter in order to help others stand up for their rights when dealing with a nursing facility. My caveat is this: ask a lot of questions, know your rights, and stand up for them; because like us, a skilled nursing facility may be the best option you have.

ONLY TWELVE HOURS AFTER WE WATCHED MARDIG WALK ACROSS the threshold toward an entirely different way of life we received the worst possible phone call. That evening, shortly after having a relaxing and enjoyable dinner with Lew, a call came from the sheriff's office. My father had disappeared from the facility! I was shocked.

As exhausted as we were from all of the events during the preceding days, we mustered up our reserves to search for him. The deputy said he had been looking for my father and was unsuccessful. Lew offered to help us. Our hearts racing, our energy depleted, we received strength from our adrenaline.

We took a few minutes to plan. Lew would take David's cell phone and go along a certain route, and David and I would go together along another route. Whoever found Mardig would call the other. I then telephoned the facility, gave them my cell phone number, and told them what we were going to do.

David and I searched everywhere. We walked into stores, a nearby hospital, and looked up and down the streets. Some people said they had seen a man who fit the description we gave; others said they had seen no one. Most were kind and offered to detain Mardig and call us if they saw him.

The search continued. During this time, we paid two visits to the facility and spoke with the administrator and management staff. It was a living nightmare which I detailed that night in my journal. Only minutes after we returned home, I wrote all the details I could remember. Something told me I should, because I might need documentation later. Also, writing helped me overcome the shock I felt over the whole situation.

Friday, January 31, 1997   12:26 a.m.

Mardig disappeared! He was last seen at about 7:15 p.m. according to the director of nurses and at 7:20 p.m. according to an Armenian aide who was with him. The aide said she was watching TV with Mardig and speaking in Armenian about the *good old days* when she got up to go get some food. When she returned, he was gone. She thought he had gone to his room.

The director of nurses said she got the call that my father was nowhere to be found at 8:20 p.m. The facility's staff discovered his disappearance at 8:00 p.m., the time they give out medications and check on all the residents. Why were we called a little after 9:00 p.m., over an hour after the facility realized he was gone?

The administrator explained that a lot of visitors leave at 8:00 p.m. and that Mardig could have gotten out among them.

David and I drove slowly along the main road toward the facility, thinking Mardig may have tried to walk home. We doubted this because it was dark, and he got disoriented easily. Still, we drove behind the church where the Adult Day Care Center meets. We noticed the lights were on and hoped to see people we knew. Another group was meeting. We asked them if they had seen an elderly man and proceeded to describe Mardig. They had not. *We were shaking with fear. We had done a good thing for my father by bringing him to California and now look what happened!* We continued driving on the busy street, carefully looking up and down the side streets. We saw nothing.

We drove to the facility and saw the sheriff's car parked in front. We talked with the deputies who were called there because of Mardig's disappearance. We asked them to advise us on how they were conducting the search. They said when a child disappears they knock on all the neighborhood doors and ask questions. They added that since my father is an adult, they could not do this. I asked what if the adult has the thinking ability of a child. They apologized and said they just did not have the resources to conduct such a search. *We didn't feel very confident about what our tax dollars could buy at this moment.*

We departed and continued our search. What we thought would take minutes was stretching to over an hour. The longer it took the more we lost hope. About two hours later we felt like giving up. *He was nowhere. What were we to do?* Suddenly, the phone rang. They found my father. He was walking in Rosamond. *This was another county! How did he get way out there?* We called Lew and asked him to meet us at the facility. We needed his support.

When we walked into the facility, the administrator and director of nurses were seated in the administrator's office. Upon entering, a strange sensation overcame me. This experience had been very scary and potentially dangerous. Yet, something didn't feel right.

The words I heard were, "I don't know if we can keep your father here." *Just like that. No discussion, nothing!*

I could not accept the administrator's position. My mind raced. I was responsible for Mardig as his attorney-in-fact. I believed the facility did not act responsibly and had endangered my father's life.

Before my father was admitted into the facility, the admissions representative and a supervisor explained their security procedures. We were shown the doors with built-in 15-second delay mechanisms. When a person first pushes on the door an alarm sounds, 15 seconds later, the lock releases, and the door opens. This is just enough time for an aide to reach the door and prevent a resident from leaving. We were told that the lobby area was monitored closely, especially when people came in and out. Furthermore, we were assured that, for the first two weeks, my father would receive a lot of attention by the staff until he adapted to and felt comfortable in his new surroundings. After he was admitted, the staff mentioned how much they enjoyed him and that he was fun to be with.

There was a breach. We were told no alarms sounded. How could Mardig leave among departing visitors, if there was someone watching at the front desk? Didn't the person at the front desk have to let visitors out?

We had learned that some visitors knew the codes which open the doors. We asked the administrator about this. She immediately assured us that visitors do not have access to the codes. Yet, in the three times that I had already visited the facility, I observed staff members openly punch in the four-digit code number. They seemed to make no attempt to hide it. Imagine all the warnings we have been given about covering our PINs when accessing an ATM or using our calling card. When the staff punched in the code number a visitor could easily see. The administrator further assured us that the codes were changed monthly.

My concern here is that we were repeatedly told the procedures and practices followed by the facility. We knew Mardig was a wanderer. We had informed the admissions representative and the social services director. They acknowledged this, and assured us that they were capable of handling wanderers. They added that other residents wander as well. *Yet, what good are procedures, if they are not adhered to?*

The director of nurses said that the nurses and aides who were responsible would be written up. Is she acknowledging fault here? I volunteered that "writing them up" or finding blame was not necessary. Finding the *cause* was imperative in order to secure the residents' safety. I think the director of nurses drew some comfort from the idea that I didn't want to punish her staff. I wanted them to carefully reexamine their procedures and take measures to ensure they were followed. When I mentioned this, the administrator agreed that it was a good suggestion and that they would look at their procedures again.

The administrator may have sensed that I meant no harm when she surprised us with her candor. She said it was difficult to manage the staff closely. She said it was hard to find quality nurse's aides. She volunteered that she didn't care about a lawsuit and was foremost concerned about residents' safety. *I had no intention to sue. What point would it serve? This was a problem with following procedures.*

David said that when we were first looking at this facility, we were told residents tried to hide in crowds of people to get out. A nurse's aide mentioned there were two or three incidents where residents got out within their first days at the facility. Prior to admitting Mardig, we were assured that the staff anticipated this kind of behavior and was prepared for it.

Just then, the administrator received a phone call. The deputies had arrived with my father. We heard loud noises and got up to look. Mardig was being escorted from the back of the facility by two aides. For such a cold winter evening he was out with only a flannel shirt and pants, plus his baseball hat. He looked disheveled. His shirt was half pulled out of his pants. One of his pants' pockets was pulled out. He felt cold to my touch and seemed irritated.

When I asked what happened, he said he didn't understand what was happening. He explained that he asked people to let him out of the front door after he had conversed with some

Armenians. Then he walked and walked. He claimed he was up for two nights, he was out without a jacket, the truck that he rode in had no heat, and he was cold. He said he was walking and walking and walking, he walked everywhere when a man saw him struggling on the side of the road and pulled up beside him. He looked inside the truck and saw a friendly looking man so he got in. He added, "We went to the place where the situation was occurring."

He was found about 11:00 p.m. We planned to call the sheriff's office to get more details.

The nurse's aides took Mardig to his room to get him settled. We returned to the administrator's office where she and the director of nurses expressed their heartfelt concern that one of them would have to stay up all night with Mardig. The director of nurses added that she did not feel safe without one of them staying.

There was nothing more to say or do. After we said our good-byes, Lew, David, and I sat in our car and talked about what happened. Lew shared his concern about the administrator's and director's apathy and unwillingness to follow their procedures.

Moments later, we saw them leaving the facility heading toward their cars. Both had their coats on, and their arms were filled with materials. I was surprised to see both of them because of their earlier comments about one of them staying up all night with Mardig. When they saw us sitting in our car (ours and theirs were the only cars in the front parking lot), they walked toward one another and talked for a few minutes, then the director of nurses drove away. The administrator returned to the facility. Lew, David, and I talked awhile longer, and then Lew went to his car and we drove away.

Later than morning, after trying to get a few hours of sleep, I tried to sort my thoughts. *I couldn't believe the administrator would have the nerve to suggest my father should leave. After everything we just experi-*

enced, the forms, the questions, the tour, and the options we reviewed; no, this was the best place for Mardig right now. I had to make sense of what was happening. I couldn't stop feeling nervous. I was under so much stress I could not eat or sleep. I was exhausted. I felt an incredible urge to document everything, just in case there was a lawsuit.

I took time to record the following on my computer. As I wrote, more details came to mind. My neck and shoulder muscles tightened as I typed quickly, trying to document everything. I was to suffer many head, neck, and shoulder aches.

10:41 a.m.

I sit here pondering, "What are my rights?" I called and left a message for the attorney and asked him to call me as I needed to know my legal rights in this particular situation.

I also called a representative at the GHCH-CARE, to report this incident—a requirement for the drug study. She seemed surprised and concerned and asked what I was going to do. She wondered if I'd be able to trust the facility. She said that they should know how to deal with people who have Alzheimer's. She added that they should realize that this was his first day and that he would try to find what was familiar. (Mardig apparently told the nurse's aide that he wanted to find his children.) The CARE representative said she would call the facility.

I took time to think about the outcome I wanted. Management needed to review their policies and adhere to them. They told us that they had ways of dealing with residents who want to leave—for example, distracting and then redirecting the woman who bangs and shouts loudly as she tries to get out the front door. So then why did they not see my father leave? The administrator's explanation yesterday was that if a nurse's aide is preoccupied on the telephone with a personal matter, she will not see Mardig leave. *Now what does this say about accountability? I can't accept this!*

I want to be assured that steps are being taken to follow the procedures the facility already has in place. I want regular updates that progress is being made to follow these procedures. This is all I ask. I am not interested in suing, nor do I believe suing for money will solve the problem. Although others may sue in a similar situation, I just want the staff to follow the procedures. *Let's get on with caring for these people who, through no fault of their own, have a disease that wreaks havoc on their minds!*

10:49 a.m.

I don't want to but I am going to call the facility now. I want to know how Mardig is doing.

11:14 a.m.

I'm keying these notes into the computer while on hold after being connected to one person, then another. I am waiting to talk with the director of nurses. First, I spoke with the administrator about Mardig and tried to learn if she knew of any residents leaving. She explained that she's worked in healthcare for 21 years prior to being the administrator of this facility since it opened. She denied knowledge of any resident accidentally leaving the facility.

When I asked what she observed about Mardig, she said she does not have medical experience and will defer to her director of nurses. She added that she did call and talk with Roberta at the VNA Adult Day Care Center. She reiterated her concern for the safety and appropriate care of the resident. Despite her comments, I am left with the nagging feeling that she does not want to accept responsibility for the facility's policies and procedures.

The director of nurses picked up the phone and said she talked with Mardig this morning because he was asleep last night when she went in to see him. (The administrator had said the same thing.) Mardig told her that he had a son who lived out of state who was married and had kids. He had a daughter, Brenda. He asked her how far back she wanted him to go when she asked him to tell her of his past. He knew he was born in Armenia. Her assessment was that he is relatively high functioning for the facility. The administrator echoed this concern, wondering whether the placement was appropriate. *A fine time to wonder!* She added that she would call the ombudsman and the State Licensing Board regarding this situation. The director of nurses then placed me on hold to take another call.

I hate holding, it's such a waste of time. Given the circumstances, I held for five minutes after which she finally returned. She said she just spoke with the CARE representative but didn't share any details.

She seemed rushed to go to an 11:30 meeting. When I offered to call back, she said, "No," and asked me to continue. I did, but I felt her lack of attentiveness. *She was simply going through the motions.* I asked her if the code numbers had been changed. She said she didn't know; that was the administrator's department. I thought it was strange that she would brush aside one of the major issues we discussed the night before. I asked her if she punched in the same code she punched in yesterday, and she hesitatingly said, "Yes." I repeated what I suggested to her and the administrator the night before, that changing the code number would be the first step to improving security. She said she'd relay the message to the administrator.

As we ended our conversation, she said to call anytime if there's anything else they could do. I took this as an insincere attempt to appear polite.

"Please change the code numbers, this is the first step," I said.

She muttered "Uh-huh."

February 6, 1997

This has actually been a living hell! If I didn't care so much I wouldn't do anything.

Well, that's just it…why get into all the formalities, legalities and regulatory stuff if we don't have to?

So then, here goes...

Tuesday the 4th I went to the caregivers' support group meeting at the facility where my father resides. It was scheduled to begin at 9:30 a.m. The social services director came in at 9:40 and apologized for being late. I listened and observed intently. This would be interesting, helpful. Moments later, the social services director was called to the door by the director of nurses. They spoke awhile, and then she returned. At a little after 10:00 a.m. I asked my first question. The social services director asked me if I had any more questions.

I said, "No." *I thought it was weird to be asked such a question in a support group setting.*

She then asked if I had any comments.

I shook my head and said, "No."

She replied, "Because you have a ten o'clock meeting."

"Excuse me?" I inquired. *People didn't even know I was planning to attend. How could I have a ten o'clock?* I asked, "With whom?"

She said there's a gentleman who wants to see me and got up and motioned for me to follow her out the door.

I asked, "Who?" By this time I had packed my notebook, gathered the stuff I had brought for Mardig and was rushing to follow her out the door.

I asked, "With whom?"

She said, "[person's name]."

I inquired, "[person's name]?"

"You don't know him?" she asked, surprised.

"Who is he?"

"He can help you in dealing with these kinds of things." Then she rushed ahead of me down the hallway and I tried to catch up (this is hard with all the residents slowly ambling through the halls).

I followed her out the front doors into the administrator's office and there, to my left, seated and looking toward the floor, was the director of nurses. To my right was a man standing by the chair where I was invited to sit. He was the corporate attorney.

I was sandbagged! How could they do this to me? And to pull me out of a support group! I tried very hard to retain my composure and didn't think to ask, "Why are you meeting with me—three on one?" I did think of saying, "I want to have my attorney present." But I didn't. I just wanted a resolution of this frustrating mess created by what I believed was their irresponsibility.

After the proper (and awkward) introductions and handshakes, I told them that I would listen to what they had to say and then say what I needed to. Afterward, I would visit with Mardig and then leave the facility to clear my head.

They ignored what I said and asked if I received their letter. "No," I said.

They said Federal Express was to deliver it Saturday.

I said, "Oh, you were the ones who sent a Fed Ex package! I got a notice from them on Monday the 3rd to sign the release so they could leave the package. I should get it today (Feb. 4th)."

The administrator looked disappointed and said she'd make a copy for me.

As I read it, I became numb. I could no longer concentrate on the content. I found myself focusing on how the letter was written. The first sentence was incomplete, commas and hyphens were needed. Strangely, I gained some strength from this.

January 31, 1997

Dear Ms. Avadian,

In regards to the admission of your father Martin Avadian to the [facility] on January 30, 1997.

Because of the incident of Mr. Avadian leaving the facility on the same night of admission, and planning to so the same today January 31, we feel that were (sic) are not able to assure the safety and security of him.

[The Facility] is a secured facility for Alzheimer's and others (sic) Dementias, and is not a locked facility. Residents retain their right to leave this facility, as in any other long term care facility.

As Mr. Avadian's DPOAHC, and legal representative, please make arrangements immediately for more suitable placement for him. Please inform us of your plans on Monday February 3.

I regret that this placement was not successful, but our main concern is the safety, security, and well being of the resident.

With regards,
[Administrator]
cc: Corporate Attorney

The letter was dated one day after the incident. *So much for coping with people who have Alzheimer's. So much for giving them a chance!*

I was dumfounded! *They assumed that this placement was "unsuccessful." "Inform us...by February 3." I had not even received the letter by then! What a way to wipe their hands clean of their responsibility! I was incensed yet afraid. I had to learn my rights.*

This is an Alzheimer's facility. They know that some residents will try to get out during their first few days there. The admissions representative assured us that during the first few weeks, they keep a close eye on new residents.

They screwed up. Plain and simple. They had articulated their procedures. They just refused to be held accountable for them. Doesn't make sense!

Before I even saw their letter, I called a few people—the sheriff's office, Mardig's doctor (their medical director) who claims the placement was appropriate given Mardig's mental ability. Now, I'm calling more—three ombudsmen, deputies, CHP (to learn more details), attorneys, and friends. I wanted to get as much information as I could and to learn my rights.

The attorney and ombudsmen assured me that one of five conditions must be met for the facility to release my father:

1. The nursing home has ceased operations.

2. The resident failed to pay.

3. The resident's presence endangers others.

4. The resident's health has sufficiently improved.

5. They cannot properly take care of the resident.

During the course of talking with people I learned details of other residents' families' issues with this facility. Despite these issues and my father's escape, I wanted my father to stay there. It was a clean facility, close to home, and it generally provided quality care.

One of the ombudsmen advised me to write a letter and send a copy to the Department of Health Services (DHS). Since I learned that the facility was being investigated, I didn't want to create any more trouble. After all, where else would Mardig live? When I hesitated, she emphatically asked me to consider what I would do if I turned on the TV and heard that another resident got out, was lost, and later found dead? How would I deal with the feeling, knowing I could have brought this to DHS's attention so as to avoid future occurrences? She added, "A fat fine would be waiting for them since they found your father all the way in Kern County!" I did what I felt was best. On February 6th I completed my written response to the letter the facility handed me.

6 February, 1997

Dear [Administrator]:

This letter is to respond to and acknowledge your letter dated 31 January, 1997 and delivered to me by Federal Express on 4 February, 1997 regarding my father, Martin Avadian.

As his Attorney-in-fact, I was assured prior to his admission that [the facility] (herein referred as: "Facility") could handle a resident with my father's needs—e.g., wandering, Sundowner's syndrome. My husband and I have been regularly assured by your staff that you routinely deal with residents who want to *get out* and that you have *creative* ways of handling them.

Upon our expressed concern to your staff regarding my father's wandering and agitation, we were informed that residents have and do try to mingle among visitors near the front door and then leave! We were assured that your staff deals with this and that your policy is to have two staff members at the front desk at all times since residents do try to get out.

Given this, you can imagine the surprise and scare we received when we learned 12 hours after his admission that he could not be found in the facility! Your staff noted he was missing at approximately 7:30 p.m. on Thursday, 30 January, 1997 and we received the call at 9:05 p.m. saying a sheriff's deputy would like to speak to us. Our first thought, given all these assurances we received, *how did he manage to get out*? Yet, when we (my husband and a close family friend) walked into your office, your initial comment was, "We don't think we can keep your father here."

A report filed by the CHP noted that my father was picked up in another county! Imagine that! Due to your negligence to follow your own clearly articulated procedures to insure the safety and security of your residents...look what happened to my father. What if another resident got out and was not as lucky as my father? (We have heard from your staff that this happens!)

In spite of this oversight, I desire to keep my father in your facility. He expresses how much he likes it there. He thinks he's been there for several years. Your staff regularly informs us of how much they enjoy him. We have been told that since this initial incident he has not tried to get out. Sure, he, like many of your other residents, will express a desire to go home. Still, we have been repeatedly told that he has not tried to get out.

I would like to be assured that you will follow your procedures—changing the access code (if you have not already done so), asking your staff to keep the access code covered when entering or leaving the facility (similar to when we use ATM machines), and keeping the front desk staffed at all times. You have a very caring staff, I am sure this was as much a scare to them as it was to you and your Corporate Attorney.

I am fully aware of my rights and if we cannot resolve this situation, I will take further steps.
Genuinely yours,

Brenda Avadian
cc: [Ombudsman]

February 6, 1997   9:46 p.m.

This is getting tiring. Instead of being able to relax, I need to continue to journal in order not to lose my memory of these things. And why? Because a few people cannot be responsible nor accountable. Because such is life. We are all interconnected, what one does impacts many. The facility's oversight led to my father's disappearance which led to the involvement of a lot of people, which led to the facility's denial due to fear of accountability and liability. *Life becomes toxic when one points the finger at someone else!*

Mardig called me this morning. He is unaware of the passage of time. Instead of days, he thinks he's been living in the facility for years. He refers to his room as "home." He said, "If you have a couple hours to throw away, come visit me as I would like to talk with you at some length."

He felt awkward talking on the phone, so we started speaking in Armenian. I reminded him he could still speak Armenian and I could understand it, so he could feel free to talk.

In Armenian he said, "They're tiring me...they are asking me a lot of questions." He said he's doing nothing there but if his being there is helpful to me, he'll stay. *The never-failing diplomat, even with Alzheimer's.*

He said the staff is friendly, smiles, and is nice. He says he keeps losing his pencils and pens. (He likes writing notes to himself. Writing little notes provides him comfort, even though he loses the paper he writes notes on. He advised me to call him a day in advance of my visit so that he would be at home, since he tends to wander a lot outside. (Meanings: *home:* his room; *outside:* the halls.) He thought that he would keep in touch with me just in case I moved or changed my phone number. He wanted to be sure we were "still connected."

Jan called David this evening to apologize for not visiting Mardig today. (She had told him she would visit my father today.) Her reason? She was afraid that the facility's staff would ask her a lot of questions.

She said she felt uncomfortable and could not face their questions today. She explained that last night they took her to a room to ask her a lot of questions. *Who is she? How does she know Mardig?* Then they asked questions about David and me. She could not easily recall the specific questions. Nonetheless, before she left yesterday, they asked her for her name and number so they could contact her if necessary. She said this would be fine. Yet today, she appeared to be affected by it. *Why would they question a visitor and nonfamily member in this way?*

Friday, February 7, 1997   1:41 p.m.
I visited Mardig today from 10:55 to 11:50 a.m. He was happy to see me. I was a familiar face in a sea of unfamiliarity in whom he could confide. Jan came about 25 minutes later and we both visited with Mardig.

He said they were putting restrictions on him. He was trying to get out and they would tell him not to or gently redirect him. *This was good!* He said he wanted to get out because he wanted to walk around the area. He was used to doing that. I reminded him of the incident when he tried that and found himself in another county. I explained he was lost and the police had to bring him back. He had no recollection of the incident.

I left. Jan stayed with Mardig for a few minutes longer.

Later, Jan called to tell me that as she was leaving, the social services director said she thought Jan was my father's daughter. *Hmmmm, this is strange. Just a week earlier, I met with this director for 45 minutes to complete my father's psycho-social assessment.* The social services director asked her to relay a message to me. *Why are my father's visitors getting this kind of treatment?*

Saturday, February 8, 1997   11:15 a.m.

Jan called and said she just got back from seeing Mardig. When she got there, she said that Mardig was lying in bed reading the newspaper. Jan brought a picture with her for Mardig to put up on his white board that the facility recently mounted for us. *Does this mean he can stay?*

Mardig said the picture might get stolen if it was put up, so he placed it in his drawer instead. The picture was one of Dave and Jan dressed in formal wear.

Jan added that Mardig commented on how handsome Dave looked. Mardig also said that "Ma was very busy taking care of the kids," and that is why she doesn't come to visit him. Mardig explained that if he loses his job, he will have to get another one to make sure that all the bills are paid.

Jan said that she just listened to him talk and that she didn't really remember anything else that he said. She ended her visit when a nurse came in and said that he had to take Mardig's vitals. She said no one asked her any questions this time and it was a very pleasant visit.

11:43 a.m.   (David's notes)

Our neighbor who cares for our cats called. I told her about the situation with Brenda's father. I keep waking up in the night thinking about Mardig at the nursing home. I wake up thinking about him and go to bed thinking about him. I think about him when I am at work and on my way to and from work. I worry that the nursing home will not treat him nicely because they think that he is too much trouble. That's all.

Days pass into weeks. David and I go on our two-week business trip while Jan looks after my father. There are no other letters exchanged between the facility and me. Time passes, and Mardig grows more used to the facility and refers to it as his home. We learn that occasionally he tries to get out, as do a number of other residents. But as far as he is concerned, he is *home*.

I have not spoken to the administrator since the incident, except for an occasional "Hello." I have not seen much of the director of nurses either. I had hoped surviving this trauma together would have given us a special bond. Despite all of this, I am satisfied that my father is *home* and that he is being well cared for.

Chapter 13

MARDIG'S FIRST VISIT HOME

A FTER MARDIG HAD BEEN AT THE NURSING FACILITY AWHILE, we wanted to bring him home for a visit. We felt like parents who want their children to visit once they've left home.

The nursing facility's staff advised us not to take him out of the facility too soon as it could disrupt his adjustment to his new *home*. So we waited. We visited him regularly. Each time we wanted to bring him home the time was not right. *When* was the right time?

We grew concerned that he may never leave the facility if we waited for the *right* time. Besides, he wanted to go out! He kept asking to go out. David and I talked about it. I raised the issue at a support group meeting. The other caregivers advised us to trust ourselves as to when the time was right to take him out. There was that answer again, *"You'll* know when the time is right."

As with some things in life, it pays to be patient. The *right* time came three months after he was admitted.

᠅   ᠅

DAVID AND I FELT UNCOMFORTABLE the day we were to bring Mardig home for a visit. We had no idea what to expect. We didn't know how he would feel, what mood he would be in, if he had enough sleep the night before, how he would behave once we bought him home. We wondered what we would do if Mardig didn't want to go back once we brought him home.

Managing a child is one thing. Managing an adult who reasons like a child is another.

We called the facility in advance and told them our plans. We asked if they could help us by making certain Mardig was dressed and shaved. This way, he'd know he was going out.

We arrived at the facility with cheerful optimism trying to hide our underlying discomfort. When we saw Mardig, he was clean-shaven and dressed. He refused to wear a shirt, preferring to only wear a T-shirt. So there he was, with his T-shirt and cream-colored, pleated cotton pants with the legs tucked into his heavy white athletic socks, and black Velcro-fastened athletic shoes.

With great enthusiasm and big smiles, we asked Mardig if he wanted to see a movie. His response did not match our energy. We explained that the movie was a video we took while in Milwaukee and that he would see people he knew—his son and daughter. He looked puzzled. We repeated what we said.

He didn't answer our question but asked if we would bring him back home (to the facility). We replied, "Of course, we'll bring you back!"

He jokingly replied, "Then I'll go...can't get a better deal than that!"

David retrieved a boldly-striped cotton shirt from Mardig's closet, which Mardig put on but refused to tuck into his pants. This was atypical for him, because he was still concerned about how he looked, but it didn't matter. We just wanted to take him out. We were nearly ready to leave when he asked, "How do I look?"

"Just great! Only one more thing. Please brush your teeth." I had debated whether to ask him to brush his teeth or not and decided it would be better if he did. I wanted to enjoy his company. I wanted to feel free to lean close to him and speak in his ear when he couldn't hear. I didn't want to have to hold my breath because his was unbearable.

He asked if his breath was really bad. He had always been forthright about such things when he perceived someone cared.

I said, "Yes," and nodded.

He said, "Okay."

I pulled out his grooming kit, handed him the toothbrush, and put a little dab of toothpaste on his brush. He sat on the edge of the bed and began brushing his teeth. Once his mouth started foaming with paste he got up. Disoriented, he tried to leave the room. I gently directed him to his bathroom, where he continued to meticulously brush his teeth and gums.

When he finished, I held the toothbrush holder for him so he could slide his brush into it. Confused, he kept placing his hand on the bottom of the container fearing his toothbrush would slide right through onto the floor. Once he put his toothbrush in, I placed the top over the bottom. By this time, he was grabbing onto the entire holder, uncertain as to what would happen. I encouraged him to let it go and then shook the closed toothbrush holder. He smiled, realizing his brush was safely inside.

These are the little things we observe when our loved ones are stricken with this dementing disease. Alzheimer's is taking its toll. I watch as my father tries harder to make sense of the things most people take for granted.

We walked out of his room and went to the front desk to sign him out. Then we walked outside. He looked at the busy street out front and asked, "Hey, which street is that?" He always wanted to have his bearings.

We got into the car and started driving to our house, which was a little over four miles away. He did not seem to be as concerned about the streets while in the car. He had lost his brand-new bifocals a few weeks prior, so he could not focus on all the things that fascinated him on the street—street names, tall trees, power lines and poles. He sat in the front seat next to David and breathed heavily with a wheezing sigh. We wondered if he had caught a cold.

As we pulled onto the street off the main avenue, he asked if this was the street to our home. We said, "Yes," and complimented him on remembering. After a few more turns, we pulled into our driveway and parked in front of the garage.

He asked, "Is this your home?"

"Yes," we said.

He got out of the car with a little help and walked up the driveway to the front walk, which was partially flooded from the lawn sprinklers. He carefully tried to walk around the flooded parts and dried his feet on the doormat.

Once inside, he didn't remember a thing. He didn't realize he had lived in this house with us for nearly six months. We gave him a chair to sit on, directly in front of the television set, and then showed him some pictures of his family—daughters, son, his house. He didn't remember from one picture to the next and had to be reminded who his children were. When we started showing the video of the home he had lived in for more than half of his life, much to our surprise, he drifted in and out of sleep. When we drew his attention to the cluttered basement where he had spent a lot of his time, he said, "It was cleaner when I left it." and "Wow, I wish I had all those tools!"

He was tired. He struggled to stay awake. We reasoned that he may have stayed awake the night before. Only an hour had passed when panic overcame him. He exclaimed, "I don't want to die! I don't want to die here! I must go home now. Take me home! I must go home now."

We turned off the television set, put on our shoes, walked out to the car, and took him *home*.

Once we pulled into the parking lot, he asked, "Is this home?"

"Yes," we said. As he followed us up the ramp to the entrance, through the lobby, and then into the section where he immediately recognized the other residents, he relaxed. He felt safe, and his concerned frown relaxed into a smile. He then walked toward his room. We followed him into his room. Without a word, he took off his shirt and pants. We assumed he was getting ready for bed. I pulled back the covers, he thanked me, and then got in bed. David helped pull the covers over him. He then asked us to turn off the lights as we left.

∾   ∾

What were we to think about what had just happened? *Our* home was no longer *his* home. His home was the facility. Perhaps this was a good thing. At first, he tried to get out. Now, he felt safe because it was his home. Still, it was a little unnerving for David and me to know that Mardig would much rather go to a relatively sterile place with a single bed in a room with two roommates, instead of being comforted in our home. Perhaps we should be thankful that he was happy living in the facility and be comforted in knowing we had made the right decision.

Chapter 14

IT'S ALWAYS SOMETHING—
THE ESTATE SALE

The late Gilda Radner played a popular character, Roseanne Rosannadana, in the late 1970s on NBC's Saturday Night Live. Roseanne was a TV news reporter who, in Gilda's words, "was not afraid to be a gross pig." During the "Weekend News Update" segment of the show, Roseanne would read viewers' mail or go on and on about one topic or another. Inevitably, Roseanne would conclude her monologue with, "It just goes to show…it's always something!"

$\mathcal{H}$ERE I SIT, WONDERING WHEN ALL OF THIS WILL END. I have wondered this many times. David and I keep trying to predict that the worst is already behind us. Not having children of our own, we can only imagine the never-ending obligations parents face. At least with children there is a future. Barring any unforeseen circumstances, children grow into adults and manage their own affairs, while their parents look on with pleasure. *At least, this is the way it's supposed to be!*

People who have Alzheimer's do not grow *up.* In fact, the most caregivers can hope for is to enjoy the small gifts, such as a smile, acknowledgment of recognition, and special moments together. Any of these things provide caregivers enough pleasure to enable them to endure. (I have written about some of these moments in Part IV.)

Juxtapose these small pleasures with the sizable responsibilities. I had to sell my parents' personal effects, donate the rest, clean, and then sell Mardig's house.

I arrived in Milwaukee first, then David arrived several days later. During this period, Mardig's affairs occupied over 200 hours of David's and my time. We averaged fifteen hours per day. Some days we only had six hours to shower, eat, sleep, and take care of our personal needs. Despite our long hours, and help from my brother and sister during the last few days, we did not finish as I had hoped

My parents saved everything. Over the years, their possessions accumulated exponentially. We felt intimidated. We rented two of the largest containers the waste disposal company offered. They measured twenty-five-feet long by eight-feet wide and eight-feet tall. During a one-and-a-half-day period in April, my sister, her husband, my brother, his girlfriend, David, and I filled both of these containers.

༈ ~

WHEN DAVID AND I FIRST WALKED INTO THE LIVING ROOM in April, we came face-to-face with boxes stacked up to our shoulders. In some places, the boxes were stacked higher than we were tall. We had not seen the fireplace for years. Upstairs, the master bedroom had long lost its wide-open feel. Against every wall were boxes stacked from floor to ceiling. Even the adjacent dressing room with *his* and *her* closets was no longer used, because the stacked boxes barely left enough space to maneuver. Once we cleared away the boxes, David was surprised to find a window in the dressing room. More boxes awaited us in my old bedroom at the opposite end of the house.

If the first and second floors were overcrowded and intimidating, the attic took us over the edge. It was an archeological find. We found baby clothes, a five-year supply of toilet paper, a life-time supply of spare light bulbs, my brother's things, Christmas lights and cards, and 100 clocks (e.g., Baby Bens). My mother must have bought these clocks at an outdoor flea market and planned to sell them at a profit.

In contrast to the attic, the basement seemed to have more space. I would soon discover this was a major deception. There were four large rooms in the basement. One room was stacked floor to ceiling with boxes and containers—Mardig's old tools, motors, and wiring.

We took these boxes outside and filled the entire backyard! Mardig accumulated two or three of the same thing, particularly, electric drills. *When he couldn't find something or forgot he had a tool, he'd buy another one.*

I did find three treasures, however. One of them was an old food scale I remembered as a child. It weighed up to twenty-five pounds. Mardig used to tell me he weighed us on this scale when we were little. I also found an old collection of cameras Mardig had accumulated. The third treasure was an old hand-crank meat grinder. He would set it up on the workbench downstairs, lay clean newspaper on the table and then my mother would grind a special cut of beef for *kuftah*. This is an Armenian raw meat mixture of finely cracked wheat, green onions, parsley, and lots of cayenne pepper. Since the rest of the family disliked raw meat, my mother and I would enjoy this fine appetizer. These treasures and memories were the rewards of the overwhelming responsibilities I had reluctantly accepted.

People who came to the house (cleaning service, estate sale administrator, real estate appraiser, real estate broker), were amazed and overwhelmed by the quantity of things my parents had accumulated. I heard a lot of comments like, "Good luck." "Hope you're not an only child." "Wow, I'm *not* envious of what you have ahead of you." "Look at these antiques!"

Each box had to be opened. We started in the sunroom where Mardig kept most of his papers. Each file had to be closely examined. Files and oversized envelopes were not labeled correctly. Important and unimportant papers were mixed together. He had made a practice of hiding things. We found important papers between the pages of old newspapers stacked in the living room. We couldn't assume anything was a pile of junk and toss it. This process alone took upwards of 100 hours for the two of us—close to half of the entire time David and I spent during this April visit. I compared this to a typical full-time job. A person could work full time for two-and-a-half weeks and only make a dent in all my father's paperwork.

As we neared the end of the sunroom, we began to hope we could complete the entire job during this visit in April. Then we found more boxes piled against a china cabinet in the living room. Just when we thought we had handled the bulk of the paperwork, much more remained.

After looking in a few boxes, I realized some of the papers were Mardig's and the rest were my brother's. Since I already had enough to do with my father's things, I certainly didn't want to spend any time on my brother's. I took everything that was his and placed it in the dining room. My brother had claimed this room for a home office during my early teens, when we stopped using it for meals. To complicate matters, Mardig had placed his things in my brother's boxes. All this had to be meticulously sorted. We would not finish this job until May.

·: ·~

A MONTH AFTER THE APRIL TRIP, I returned alone to Milwaukee to finish clearing out my parents' personal effects. I hoped my sister and brother would help again. David had started a new job and could not fly back with me, and this would be the last time we would be going through my parents' things. I had to make arrangements for an estate sale (I'd never had one before) and to have the house cleaned (once the house was cleared out). After paying nearly $800 for a commercial/industrial dumping service, I learned that the city's Department of Public Works would have picked up the trash for free, since my father owned the house. Property taxes help finance special trash pickups in Milwaukee.

I called my sister and brother to persuade them to help. While I waited to hear from them, I continued processing Mardig's seemingly endless papers. All of his important papers were sent to California. David and I spent time processing these, and we still had not finished. It seemed the more we looked, the more we found. The trip in May would prove no different. *There was still too much stuff to go through!*

There I stood. In each direction I turned, there was more *stuff*. My efforts were not making a dent. I grew increasingly overwhelmed and was feeling hopeless. There were all those boxes in the upstairs bedroom that we didn't finish processing in April. I was near tears.

No one from my family would help me on this second trip. Could I just turn my back on this? Here I was, my father's POA. What if I threw everything away, and there were valuables—e.g. savings bonds, cash? Am I responsible? There was just too much to do. I didn't bargain for this! David and I just wanted to help Mardig. The task of managing his affairs was killing me. If I stuck with it, I would grow from the experience. I would learn things I would not otherwise know. Only those who suffer true hardships really grow in life.

I was trying to look at the positive side. Yet, I grew increasingly frustrated and started getting angry with my entire family.

I hated this! Why did I have to do all this? Why wasn't my brother helping me? After all, he'd lived in the house for forty-five years, rent free! What kind of person uses his parents so much and doesn't repay them with at least a minor sense of obligation? He never called when Mardig came to California. Mardig left Milwaukee in September, and it was January when I asked my sister again, "Have you heard from [our brother]?" Neither of us had heard from him! What was I doing here, taking care of all this when I was the youngest child and the first to leave the house? Why didn't my parents take care of all this stuff?

I hated their irresponsibility…their procrastination…their greed to accumulate so much. Why wasn't my sister here? I should just throw all this away. To hell with it! They don't care. My father never took the initiative to arrange his matters. After all, didn't I do what I set out to do? I brought him out to California to care for him because I knew he would not survive the Wisconsin winter.

So here I was, among my parents' things…all those things they kept from me because they didn't want me to know what they had. And here I was taking care of it all. *Is this the kind of fate life hands us?* I was amazed at what my mother packed! She and Mardig desired to move to the West Coast. They wanted to enjoy the warm climate and start a new life. Yet my mother had packed all her old things to take with her—old clothes; sewing supplies, including print fabrics from the 1960s and 1970s; even plastic bags and toilet paper. *If you wanted to start a new life, why would you take so much of the life you wanted to leave behind?*

It amazes me how we think a move to a new geographic location is get-ting away from it all and starting anew. Yet, if I bring all my old bag-gage, it's still the same old me, just a different place. The person must change, not the place, to start anew.

It was very sad to think of the way my mother meticulously packed the things she planned to take with her. There was so much. Among the things we found were thirty pairs of scissors! What would we do with all of them? Each was carefully wrapped in tissue paper and then bound with string. That April evening, a few days before David and I returned to California, my sister, brother, and I agreed to take a few items of her clothing which reminded us of her. The rest, we had to toss, sell, or give away.

The pleasant side to all my loneliness and self-pity during this May trip was quite a surprise. Whereas my brother and sister were not involved, except for those few days in April; my brother's girlfriend, whose family just went through a similar cleaning out process when her mother died, empathized and offered to help me. She cared a lot for my brother and wanted to know his family better. There was only one minor inconvenience—she did not have a car. I offered to drive her, but she preferred to have my brother bring her to the house instead. Mardig's house was fifteen miles away from where they had recently moved.

While she was with me, she worked hard and proved to be invalu-able. I couldn't thank her enough. She would get embarrassed at all my "thank you's." She was such a wonderful, kind, and caring person. She also shared some compassionate insights about my brother—the human side that I had long overlooked because we had grown apart. It was with her that I sat in the master bedroom and finished going through my mother's things. It was with her that I shared many mem-ories of my childhood.

Sharing these memories with her was hard because I knew how much nicer it would have been to hear my brother's and sister's recol-lections of our childhood, as I did in April when we spent an evening in the master bedroom going through some of Ma's things.

I remember we told stories, playfully modeled clothes, and ate take-out pizza in the master bedroom while watching videos of Mardig that David and I had brought in anticipation of such an occasion. It was an evening that ended with my brother and sister thanking me for taking on this difficult job and bringing us together.

That evening, my brother broke down and cried, even though Ma had died four years earlier. I didn't know what to think or feel when I heard him crying in his bedroom. I rarely saw him show emotion. Through the years, I grew accustomed to the more hardened and uncaring side of him. I experienced a self-centered man whenever I talked with him. My hunch was he had not yet faced his grief over Ma's passing.

Ma and he had the closest relationship in our family, so it was ironic that neither he (nor my sister) was present at her funeral, if you could call it that.

I remember I called my brother to get him involved, and asked his advice on the style of urn he thought my mother would like. His advice, "You take care of it. I trust you. I'm busy."

I couldn't understand how he could be so irresponsible. He'd promise to come to the house at an appointed hour and never showed. Like my sister, he gave one excuse after another about how busy he was. I grew tired of their excuses. *I gave up my career to handle this for the past eight months! I was just asking them for one week!*

On two occasions my brother promised to pick up his girlfriend at a given time, and didn't. Despite my repeated offers to drive her home, she declined. My brother had said his home address and phone number were none of my business, so I did not pressure his girlfriend. I was grateful that he brought her to the house.

The first time he didn't come as promised, she asked if she could spend the night at the house. During the years she had known my brother, she said she had never been in the house alone. She thought it would be nice to see what it was like to spend a night there by herself. There was no phone, no food, none of the comforts of home. We looked for some old clothes for her to change into, since she had not come prepared to spend the night. In my mind, she was roughing it, but she wanted to.

The second occasion was the day of the estate sale. My brother promised to come at 1:00 p.m. to help. I could not sleep much the night before and was up by 5:00 a.m. I was tired. All of my energy was spent. It was a long day. After waiting, hungry, and tired, my brother's girlfriend and I left Mardig's house at 6:30 p.m. and went to my brother-in-law's to make a few phone calls. She called my brother on his pager and left a message with his answering service, which had instructions to contact him immediately. The disappointment of waiting was wearing on us. We sipped beers to offset our hunger and dampen our anger (mostly mine). At 9:45 p.m., after enduring constant stomach growls and feeling shaky from lack of food, I suggested we have dinner. We decided on a Greek restaurant near her home. It was shortly before midnight when I took her home. I had a hard time keeping my eyes open all the way back to my in-laws, where I was staying.

Without her help, I would not have been able to complete all of the tasks. Everything was just too overwhelming and looked increasingly insurmountable each step of the way. Her interest and encouraging words helped me get through the last phase of my major responsibilities in Milwaukee as Mardig's POA.

⌐   ⌐

I GUESS WE FIND FAMILY WHERE WE CAN IN DIFFICULT TIMES. We were very private during my upbringing. While attending grade school, we were forbidden to tell our friends what our father did for a living. I never understood why. My mother drummed it into my head. "It's none of anyone's business. If someone asks say, 'I don't know.'"

I was to be reminded of this many years later while working for a defense contractor. I received a security clearance and then sat through special program briefings. "If anyone asks, just say, 'I don't know,'" each program security representative would advise.

Now I was sharing my family history with my brother's girlfriend, drawing comfort from her kindness and understanding, and from her empathy and genuine interest. She became my family for the time being.

In addition to her, other unexpected gifts replaced the sadness in my heart. I grew closer to Mardig's brother. This was important to me, since I did not know my father's side of the family. Misunderstandings between family members prevented us from being very close throughout much of my childhood. Nonetheless, while I was in Milwaukee, my uncle and aunt helped as best they could. My uncle has Parkinson's disease and is legally blind. He cannot walk very well and needs a wheelchair. We talked a lot by telephone. They invited me to stay with them in their beautiful home in Lake Forest, Illinois. I took them up on their invitation on several occasions.

Each time I'd visit, I stayed in a bedroom suite, complete with bathroom, walk-in closet, phone, television, and king-sized bed. *This was better than a fine hotel!* Plus, I ate home-cooked meals, spent time talking with family—my aunt and uncle, their children, and grandchildren.

We reminisced about my father's and uncle's childhood and looked at my uncle's collection of pictures. I was getting spoiled. At the end of each visit, I found it increasingly difficult to return to Mardig's house in Milwaukee to finish all the work that remained.

Besides Mardig's childhood pictures, none of which I'd ever seen before, another unexpected gift was the stack of letters Mardig had written to my uncle while he served in World War II. My uncle brought all of them back when he returned from the war. I read each one, and then my uncle arranged to have copies sent to me. What a treasure!

Knowing how I dreaded going back to work, they offered to visit during the estate sale. I was genuinely moved when they showed up. Seeing I was exhausted, they insisted I get away for a little while to eat lunch. I asked my brother's girlfriend to keep her eye on things while I took a brief break with my aunt and uncle.

The estate sale was physically tiring and, much to my surprise, emotionally draining as well. Seeing my parents' things go out the door in strangers' hands was difficult. "What did they pay for that?" I asked the estate sale administrator repeatedly. The prices didn't make sense. Things that should have sold inexpensively captured higher prices.

Things that deserved higher prices sold relatively inexpensively. And then there was the issue of the administrator herself.

Could I trust the estate sale administrator? There was something about her that didn't seem right. I couldn't really explain why, but I felt a need to be present. Perhaps it was that she tried to impress me with her achievements. Then again, I had never experienced an estate sale before. David and I never went to garage sales, flea markets, and the like. So, it may have been the uncertainty of the whole thing. Still, I could not have accomplished disposing of all these things alone nor could I have arranged to sell the house so quickly at an acceptable price. My suspicions, however, would be validated later when she did not uphold our agreement.

When we returned to Mardig's house, I was surprised to see my sister. She also was surprised when she saw our aunt and uncle. We sat in their Chevy Suburban for a while and talked. Later my aunt and uncle left, and my sister stayed.

My sister started asking a lot of questions about the estate sale. She made highly critical comments, telling me how things should be done and for what they should sell. She even challenged the estate sale administrator, who later told me she was offended by my sister's remarks. I didn't mind this too much given my concerns about the administrator; yet, my sister showed no initiative to help earlier. So I was not really receptive to her *after-all-the-hard-work-was-done* criticism. My sister and I began arguing. I was tired and lost patience with her. I told her I thought she was selfish and self-centered. I told her that she never thought about all the tasks I had to accomplish with Mardig's house…that she was thinking narrowly about her life…that she never contemplated the ludicrousness of a person traveling so far to take care of something a person who lived only five blocks away could handle. Needless to say, she walked out the door, got into her car, and did not speak to me again.

◆   ∾

DAYS LATER, THE UNSOLD ITEMS WERE DONATED, the house was sold, and I had a few regrets. I knew in my heart that if my sister and brother were involved, we would have done better. I had invited them many times. Sure, we would have quarreled. We're siblings. But if we got through it, we would have shared so many memories and would have been better as a family for it.

There remained the issue of the agreement between the estate sale administrator and me. She wanted me to immediately send her a finder's fee for finding a buyer of the house. Since the house had not yet been sold, I could not justify sending her this fee. I refused and this initiated a number of long-distance telephone arguments regarding the definition of "finder."

Concerned whether I was being fair, I called to ask the real estate broker who helped me earlier. She informed me that only those who held a real estate license could legally collect fees for *selling* or *finding a buyer* for a house. The estate sale administrator did not have such a license. Perhaps she was concerned about breaking the law.

Nevertheless, I held my ground and waited until the house closed escrow to send her the finder's fee.

The second part of our agreement was that she would send me a *signed* copy of her appraisal. I still have not received it.

These annoying details made me thankful that this estate sale experience was now behind me.

∾   ∾

AFTER ALL I'D BEEN THROUGH DURING THE LAST EIGHT MONTHS, I thought the worst was over. No more fifteen to eighteen-hour days trying to do a job which I later learned takes months. From now on, I could visit Milwaukee and enjoy myself. In California, only little details remained. I would easily fit them into my schedule. I could take care of *my* businesses which had suffered due to my neglect.

Chapter 15

IT'S ALWAYS SOMETHING— SEXUALITY

During a television interview, Gilda Radner explained that her father used to say, "It's always something." So, she used it in Saturday Night Live. Sadly, this was also the title of her book, which chronicled her fateful struggle with ovarian cancer.

1 RETURNED TO CALIFORNIA AND LEARNED THAT MARDIG WAS exhibiting inappropriate sexual behavior. *What does this mean?* Although it is common for some people with Alzheimer's to exhibit sexual behaviors, it's potentially embarrassing for family members and caregivers. *But my father?*

My father was the ideal diplomat, a gentleman. Even though his teen years were partially spent on the streets of Chicago, he had a polite respect for others. I recall many lectures during my childhood when I was taught how to treat people. In recent years, he and I talked on the phone about how to relate with people. I would raise a particular work problem, and his advice always came around to respecting others, especially those in higher positions than me. *How much of his advice I followed is another matter.*

Regarding sexuality, he was very close-lipped. He would not tell dirty jokes. As kids, our friends asked us if we knew any dirty words in Armenian. When we asked him, he would not tell us. He wouldn't even tell us once we were adults! I viewed him as a discreet and proper man regarding sexual matters.

So it is in this context that I was alarmed by this report of his behavior. In June, during a quarterly review at the Alzheimer's facility where Mardig lives, his behaviors were slowly revealed to me.

I am told these review sessions are mandated by the federal government and monitored by the State Licensing Board. They usually consist of a person representing social services, nursing, activities, nutrition, and more. I was impressed with the dedication of personnel to take time out of their already burdened schedules to conduct these meetings.

Still, I sensed an adversarial tone to these meetings (this was my second one). *Could it be because my father established his reputation on the first day of his admittance by walking out the front door, only to be found lost and confused in the Mojave Desert?*

Instead of "How can we work together for the common good?" these meetings felt more like, "We will give you this information, and we urge you to do what we say." Now, this may just be me. And I know that Mardig was a handful for the facility when he first arrived. So this, by itself, may cause a *bit* of a problem.

Still, it's one of those situations where you try to work with people whose livelihoods involve taking care of your loved one. You want a healthy exchange of ideas.

But for one reason or another, management seemed to have their own ideas. If I didn't agree with them, I was perceived as being difficult. If I gave them feedback (e.g., "My father's glasses are still missing, can you please find them?" "My father's gums are getting infected, and his front top teeth are looking grayer. Are you making sure the aide brushes them at least once a day?"), I feared they would find little ways to make life difficult for Mardig, or worse, remove him from the facility for a "legitimate" reason. This has happened! I've learned of two instances where a resident was removed. I am told there was little the families could do.

On the other hand, if I was afraid to give feedback, what would happen? My father might not be cared for the way he should be. "It shouldn't be this difficult," I kept telling myself. But it was. I still don't know how to proceed. It seems that for $120 per day—nearly

$44,000 per year—in a three-person room, my father should be cared for *just a little more.*

They begin by telling me that Mardig hasn't changed much.

This catches me off guard because I've noticed a big change in his ability to recall who I am. He doesn't realize I am his daughter. Sometimes, I am his son. Most of the time, I am a familiar face that makes him feel comfortable and safe, a person who will rescue him from his perceived troubles. On rarer occasions, I am one of his parents, his "Ma" or "Pa," gender doesn't make a difference. I ask the committee what they mean by "Mr. Avadian has not changed much."

Another representative tells how my father continues to wander and how he got out of the facility a couple of times with visitors who were leaving. *Didn't we cover this subject in detail with the administrator and director of nurses when Mardig first got out? We were told many residents pose this problem to varying degrees, initially. Months after this meeting I would personally witness one female and two male residents making repeated attempts to leave. One male resident made it all the way out into the parking lot and had to be coaxed inside by an aide. To my knowledge, however, none have come close to "The Great Escape" engineered by my father. Even though I can laugh about it now, it was nerve-wracking then. So, given the gravely serious potential consequences, I decide to offer some common-sense suggestions once more.*

I suggest they monitor the doors and urge visitors to be careful when they leave. Although my suggestions are unsolicited, I stand to demonstrate how we can open and then close the door behind us to make sure no one slips through. I think this is unnecessary and should be common sense, but I proceed because Mardig's life depends on it. One of the committee members is not even looking. No one is taking notes. *Of course not! Why should they? This is common sense!* I add that they should post a sign asking visitors to be sure to close the door behind them as they leave, so residents cannot leave accidentally. I demonstrate how I look behind me as I pull the door closed to make sure it is latched. *I am convinced my words are falling upon deaf ears, so I sit down.*

They tell me that my father no longer asks for pencils, pens, maps, or phone books. He used to take notes and look up banks and people's names he remembered in the phone book. He was an avid note taker and kept detailed journals. After he lost his glasses, his desire to read and write waned.

They explained Mardig still walks around "on a mission." They tell me he resists their attempts to redirect him. I take the liberty to offer one more unsolicited suggestion. *You'd think I'd learn my lesson from the lack of attention I received for the first one. I try to explain how they need to patiently "connect" with a person before trying to redirect him/her. I am met with equal inattention.*

One representative tells me that my father organizes other people's drawers. She explains that he is up all night wandering, setting off alarms (when he tries to exit a door), disturbing residents during sleeping hours by rummaging through their drawers. *Wow, I remember how this was when he lived with us. We could not sleep the whole night uninterrupted.*

It wasn't until I prompted them for more updates, that I nearly fell under the weight of what Mardig had been doing. The representatives started fidgeting and looking awkwardly away. They started slowly. One representative said, "Your father relieves himself inappropriately." Then she paused for my reaction.

Who comes prepared for this? I thought back to January when he was still living with us. He would use the bathroom, and he'd miss the toilet altogether. We'd later find urine on the toilet and down the sides, on the vanity and bathtub, we'd see puddles on the floor, and stains on his clothes. Wanting to be sure I knew what they were speaking of, I asked, "What do you mean?"

"He relieves himself in the corridors."

"Oh really?" *I imagine how difficult this must be for them. I remember how much effort he required while he was living with us. This facility is kept very clean. In fact, it is continually cleaned, if the powerful smell of cleaning solution is any indication.*

"What else does he do?"

The representatives looked at one another and then one spoke, "He exposes himself."

I try to hide my surprise. In my mind, I know that this is natural for the state he's in. He is not aware of the things he is doing because his brain is being destroyed by this disease. I really cannot fault him. I can only accept what is. "Really? How so?" I ask as calmly as I can muster.

"Well, we saw him holding himself in the dining room."

"Hmmmm." *I try to keep a straight face while fighting off my disbelief.* I paraphrase for clarification, "You mean he unzips his pants and holds himself?"

"Yes," comes the quick confirmation.

"Have you seen him do this?" I ask the social services director who responded affirmatively.

"No, I got it off the report." *The nursing staff maintains weekly reports on each resident. In Mardig's case, these reports have become a daily occurrence.*

"Has anyone seen this?" I ask the group.

"Yes," the activity representative replies.

"What did he do?"

"Well, he was standing in the dining room holding himself."

"Then what?"

"Well," she hesitated, "he was exposing himself to the other residents."

I just couldn't imagine my father doing this.

"What did they do?"

"Oh, some got irritated, others ignored him."

A mischievous and naughty thought popped in my mind, "My father can't even be a 'turn-on' in an Alzheimer's facility!"

"What did you do?" I asked.

"Well, I walked in front of him and asked him to put himself away. I told him that this behavior was inappropriate."

"Did he understand?"

"Yes, I suppose."

"What did he do?"

"Martin said he couldn't. He smiled sheepishly and said he was hard." *Wow, this is getting embarrassing. My father...?*

We were smiling awkwardly at this time. "So what did you do?"

"I redirected him away from the other residents and helped him zip his pants."

"Wow," I exclaimed and then shared with them a little about my father's nature. I described the way he was and how surprised he'd be if he knew this was what he was doing. This behavior is so foreign to the way he lived his life. He was quite the gentleman.

They explained such behavior is typical for some of the residents who were sexually proper. I heard from residents' family members that one woman routinely took her clothes off and paraded up and down the halls of the facility. Another man regularly brought women into his room…which lead me back to my father. "What else does he do?" I asked.

Again, they glanced at one another, as if to ask, "Should we tell her?"

"He urinated in a cup and then offered it to one of our female residents."

"Hah, like an offering!" I exclaim, trying desperately to lighten up the heaviness in the room.

Some chuckle, the rest remain serious. "What else does he do?"

"He tries to bring women into his room."

"Have you seen this?" I ask the representative who tells me this.

"No, but I've read the reports and one of the aides said she went into his room and saw him with another woman."

I think it is nice that Mardig is trying to enjoy himself in the company of a woman. However, given his mental state and that of the other residents, I wonder about the risks of physical injury and emotional pain. A very young child catching her parents making love may see the act as painful. I share this with the committee. They seem to accept these comments graciously.

I think about how awful this would be for the husbands of female residents. For example, I imagine if Jonathan, who visits his wife frequently, would walk in and see my father with his wife.

"Is this like taking care of children?" I wonder. I mean, we have to take seriously what our children do. We can't ignore it. "If Mardig, who

granted me Durable Powers of Attorney for Healthcare and other mat-
ters (financial, etc.), behaves inappropriately, am I responsible?"

The committee then advises me to speak with the director of nurses who will urge me to have Mardig seen by a psychiatrist. A *psychia-*
trist? How can a psychiatrist help someone with Alzheimer's? I ask her
this, and she says my father's mental condition needs to be evaluated,
as does his need for possible medications. *My father has Alzheimer's.*
What is there to be evaluated? The psychiatrist will prescribe *drugs.*

In my thinking, this is the beginning of the end.

·:   :·

MARDIG WAS EIGHTY-SIX YEARS OLD and took no medications. This was
highly unusual for a person his age. So, I struggled with thoughts of
getting him started, polluting his body, and balancing multiple medications. During the last years of my mother's life, her dosage had
increased to seven pills, four times a day. The chemical reactions
among the pills, which were supposed to help her enlarged heart function, played havoc with her mind. *Sure, first it's one pill, then two, and*
then more, as my father slides downhill.

·:   :·

I RAISE THE MEDICATION ISSUE at our weekly caregiver support group
sponsored by the VNA Adult Day Care. Some of the members dis-
agree that prescription drugs are the beginning of the end. They argue
that whatever helps my father function comfortably with this disease is
best. "No use in letting him be tortured as he tries to live day to-day.
Besides, his aggressive behavior may be a risk to the other residents,
and he may have to be removed from the facility." This last comment
strikes terror in my heart. I prefer Mardig to be close to my home
where I can see him often.

The worst may not yet be over. "It's always something."

I'm afraid. If we don't get medications for Mardig, the director of
nurses and her staff may make a case for removing him. I believe they
are being much too hasty, jumping to a quick solution for a situation
that is common among people with Alzheimer's. First, one pill, then

another, and soon Mardig will be a *zombie!* My mind is racing with thoughts of what to do next. *They can't force my father to take drugs.*

I call Mardig's doctor and ask his opinion. I express my concern about starting him on medications. He seems to understand and tells me he will be visiting the facility (as he does weekly) to check up on his patients. *He sees a great number of the residents. I don't know how many, but he is there often enough that the former admissions representative introduced him to me as their medical director.* He assures me that he will discuss my father's situation with them.

I am left with the same thoughts I had when I first chose him to be Mardig's doctor. If he's regarded as their medical director, won't he have a conflict of interest? Won't he be more inclined to represent the facility's interests than Mardig's? On the other hand, if he sees a lot of patients, I can depend on his regular visits and greater knowledge of what happens to people with this disease. I was told that not all doctors are willing nor do they routinely come to the facility to check on their patients. This was my dilemma as I waited to hear from him.

I went to the support group meeting and spoke of my concerns, particularly about this doctor's potential conflict of interest. Roberta, who also served as our facilitator, encouraged me to call the doctor and share my concerns.

With her encouragement, I called the doctor's office a few days later. *I had expected he would call me after seeing Mardig since I had expressed so much concern.* Surprisingly, he told me the same thing that the director of nurses said, "Have a psychiatrist see your father." I asked him if there were any other options. He said I could have Mardig moved to another place where he could receive one-on-one care. I asked if he knew of any place nearby.

He said, "No."

I asked, "Are these my only two options?"

He said, "Yes."

I was suspicious. Did the staff at the facility talk with him and suggest he strongly recommend that my father see a psychiatrist and then be medicated? I did not want to go down this path.

A thought occurred to me. I wanted to talk with him about Mardig's expressed wishes regarding life-support. I had heard too many stories of the nightmares resulting from a loved one being placed on life-support because the doctor or hospital was unaware of a living will. I did not want this to happen to Mardig.

When I called the doctor's office again, I asked to speak with him. I was going to talk with him about Mardig's wishes, but when he picked up the telephone, my brain froze. I told him I wanted to set an appointment to discuss patient philosophy with him. As soon as I said this, I realized it was the wrong thing to say. My abrupt request to discuss *patient philosophy* may have implied dissatisfaction with his care. I grew nervous and couldn't think of a way to retract my statement.

Mardig's doctor suggested that if I wanted another physician it was okay with him.

I immediately backed off in surprise. I knew what I had done. However, I didn't think he would take such offense at my request. I stammered and said I just wanted to *talk* with him.

He said I could talk with him while we were on the telephone.

His reactions were not reducing my nervousness. I said I would feel better in a face-to-face meeting.

He seemed to resist the idea.

After my repeated insistence, he grudgingly agreed to meet with me.

I told David about this, and we considered whether there were cultural and/or gender issues here. We agreed David would take time off from work to accompany me to this meeting, just in case this doctor had difficulty respectfully acknowledging concerns expressed by a female.

I didn't want to let culture get in the way of my father's health. David took time off work so we could talk with Mardig's doctor. We met for forty-five minutes and had a great discussion about the issues (medications, desire to stay at the facility, and life support). The doctor said he would monitor Mardig's behavior. He urged us to have Mardig seen by a psychiatrist. We agreed to take this route if his inappropriate sexual behaviors continued. The doctor appeared to accept this. David and I felt, for the moment, that we finally saw eye-to-eye with the doctor.

~: ~

DILEMMAS. If it's not one thing, it's another. Emotionally, all of this was very draining. All this thinking exhausted us—the sleepless nights, tossing and turning, trying to make sense of something we knew little about. *Why did it have to be this way?*

Other caregivers gave me strength by complimenting me on caring so much. They commented on my attention to detail in looking after my father's affairs. Some suggested that my questions intimidated others. Perhaps I get my questioning skill from Mardig. He was an avid questioner—the original inquiring mind. He knew his subjects well.

So many of us go through life knowing very little about many things. Everything my father learned, he tried to know in-depth. I often express it this way, *we can either learn one inch deep about a mile wide or a mile deep about one inch wide.* I prefer the latter because asking questions and then really listening is a discipline that can be applied inch-by-inch as the miles add up in our lives.

~: ~

FORTUNATELY, THINGS TURNED OUT NICELY. Mardig stopped displaying inappropriate sexual behavior. This meant that we did not have to have him seen by a psychiatrist, and he would not be placed on any medications for this behavior.

~: ~

LOOMING OVERHEAD, THE EVER-PRESENT ISSUE: *When am I going to get on with my life? I wonder to what extent my sister and brother would have gone out of their way to care for Mardig.* Other caregivers continue to encourage me with their heartfelt compliments.

"You are such a devoted daughter. Regardless of how you may be getting behind in your life right now, you will be glad you cared for your father."

"You won't regret this."

"Your father is so fortunate to have you."

"I wish you were my daughter. When I need care, I wish you would be there."

PART IV

Memories

Chapter 16

WE WILL LAUGH ABOUT THIS IN
YEARS TO COME

*W*HENEVER WE ENCOUNTER CERTAIN CHALLENGING life experiences, we comfort ourselves with that old phrase, "We will laugh about this in years to come." Well, there are a few of these moments when caring for a loved one with Alzheimer's.

～ ～

MIRROR MIRROR ON THE WALL...

A few funny incidents David and I recall occurred in front of a mirror. There were two mirrored closet doors in Mardig's bedroom. A few weeks after he came to live with us, we overheard him talking in his bedroom. Since only the three of us were home, David and I quietly walked to his bedroom and stood at his open door. We could barely contain our laughter when we saw Mardig standing directly in front of one of the mirrored doors, having a conversation with his reflection!

We looked at each other and laughed quietly, then continued watching my father grow increasingly irritated at the unresponsive image in the mirror. We walked back into the living room and tried to make sense out of what we had seen. This was so different from our everyday experiences; we didn't know what to do.

This behavior continued over the weeks. Mardig would call us into his bedroom and show us the person who was mimicking him. He'd express how irritating it was. Again, we didn't know what to think. He'd say, "Look at him! All he does is mimic me and doesn't answer my questions. He looks stupid." *To think he was speaking of himself— his reflection.*

We tried a few things, including using a videocamera to help him understand the difference between his physical self and his image reflected by a mirror or on the television. He could not grasp the difference. We'd touch him and ask him what he felt. He'd acknowledge our touch. Yet, while touching him, when we asked him to look at his and our images in the mirror or on the television, he couldn't make that leap. He understood the difference between David's and my images on TV and in the mirror, but he couldn't comprehend his own reflected image. The man in the mirror or on TV was someone else.

Mardig went so far as to suggest we contact the station manager because there was someone on television who looked exactly like him. "Hey, you or David need to write a letter to the…the station…to the manager of that channel…which channel is that? There's a guy on there that looks just like me. They can research it."

As I ran the camera for these extended periods, we tried to reason with him. I thought, "This would be a funny submission to *America's Funniest Home Videos.* The poor guy, he had no idea. Could this video help an Alzheimer's research organization understand how victims of Alzheimer's think? How they process information?

Several weeks passed before David came up with the brilliant idea of re-installing the closet doors with the mirrored sides facing in. He even got Mardig to help him re-install them one weekend. It didn't do much for the room's decor, but it certainly gave my father peace of mind.

～　～

David is losing his mind.
While I was in Dallas on business, David sent me the following two e-mails, which I accessed with my laptop.

Brenda,

I think I am losing my mind. I could have sworn that I had your father's tax papers, so let me ask you, do I? Or are they in the office closet on top of the box? I'm sorry for asking this, but I swear that your father is repeatedly coming into our bedroom at night and I think he may have taken some of his papers.

Last night he got up at 3:30 a.m. and started shaving, he walked around the house for a while, and then went back to bed. I have to be awake to make sure that he doesn't turn on any gas. He turned on the gas valve to the fireplace the other day and I caught it right away.

But last night was weird. I was half awake and half asleep, and I KNOW that something got on the bed with me. It seemed like it was the size of a cat, but at the same time, it was like someone or something was patting me, trying to figure out what the shape of my body was. I clearly remember my thoughts while this was happening, "This has happened to me many times before." I wasn't scared at all. I also remember thinking that whatever was on me or feeling me had the ability to make me immobile—I truly could not move although I was aware. I remember trying with all my might to get whatever it was off of me. It was like a contest of wills.

I won! But I broke free with such a force that everything on the bed went flying across the room.

After this happened, I was so convinced that something or someone was by the clothes' valet that I grabbed the flashlight to see. Of course, nothing was there. But I know something was on the bed. I would bet my life on it. I am starting to wonder if your father is moving stuff without me knowing it (and without him knowing it too).

I just wanted to share this experience with you because it was bothering me all day and probably will for the rest of the week. Now, I can't find what I did with the tax papers. So I am starting to think I have Alzheimer's.

∿   ∿

DAVID BREAKS HIS TOES.

Three days later, David sent the following e-mail. Sally was helping take care of Mardig, and she had invited David and Mardig to dinner...

Brenda dear,

Dinner at Sally's was nice. Except Mardig was ornery during dinner. He said he wanted something to eat after he finished dinner but wasn't going to tell me what he wanted. He said I had to figure it out for myself. It wasn't a toothpick, it was bread. He said he needed bread to drink his soda. He really likes Wonder Bread. Amazing!

When we got home, he wanted to go straight to bed. While I was helping your father get ready for bed, I heard a noise in the living room. I knew the cats had just finished eating so I thought the noise was them. I ran into the living room because I knew Sev would try to pee on the drape. I forgot to lift my foot up over the concrete base of the fireplace and heard a loud crack in my foot. My middle two toes are now swollen, and I have trouble walking.

So let's see, I live in a house with three cats who will try to pee on anything when a human is not in the room, one 86-year old who gets lost in the house, who can't see very good, can't think very good, and can't hear. Now, I'm a cripple and I have to somehow supervise all the 'animals' in the house (at all hours of the day), then I have to drive 83 miles to work and come home and hear the same group of 20 questions about 30 times.

Boy, life is wonderful, and I feel EXCELLENT! I say this all in humor. I am getting by OK.

Love, David

The following day, David went to the doctor and had an x-ray of his foot. The crack he heard was indeed a bone breaking. He was given a special shoe to wear and told it would take six weeks to heal.

~: ~

PAUL IS BURNING DOWN THE HOUSE.
During one of our support group meetings, Paul shared the following personal experience:

My wife likes ham and beans. I was preparing some in a large Dutch oven so I could give her some when I went to visit her in the convalescent home.

I went to a restaurant to have some breakfast. While eating, I heard sirens and saw fire trucks race by. I thought, "Gee, I wonder whose house is burning down?"

I finished breakfast and headed home to go pick up the ham and beans to surprise my wife. As I approached, I saw a lot of emergency vehicles on my street! I drove forward until I reached **my house** and realized that they had come to my house! I wondered what happened.

My neighbor came by and explained. He heard my fire alarm go off and he called the fire department. They came in through the back—I had left the patio door open. They found the stove still on and the ham and beans cooked to a crisp in the Dutch oven.

Stupid me! I had left the stove on when I went to breakfast!

⌁   ∾

I DROVE INTO THE CLOSED GARAGE DOOR.

No matter what our age, all of us experience moments when we're thinking about something else and not concentrating on what we are doing. I'm in my late thirties, and yet on three occasions I was so preoccupied with how I was going to handle my father's affairs, that I backed my car out of the garage *before* the door was open! If I tally up the damages; there were two power antennas at $120, two damaged garage doors at $850 (we changed the door only once), and damage to my Miata's flawless exterior ($750).

⌁   ∾

THE CHILDHOOD BULLY RETURNS.

Sometimes, I think about certain people from my childhood. They come to mind every now and then, and I wonder what happened to them.

When I was in fifth grade, the class bully would approach me on the playground and taunt me. I'd try to ignore her, but she'd hit me. I'd walk away, but she and a group of girls would follow me. This happened repeatedly. One time, I couldn't take it anymore. She hit me hard, and I began to cry. I was afraid and embarrassed.

As the years passed, I would wonder, "What happened to her? Is she a successful professional somewhere? Did she drop out of school? Did she have children? Where does she live?"

The estate sale was about to begin and I wanted to capture everything on videotape beforehand. The estate sale administrator's assistant agreed to videotape me while I walked around and described everything. We started outside on the sidewalk. A wide-angle shot included the house with me standing in the foreground. Just as I began saying a few words about the house and the park across the street, a van pulled up. In a matter of seconds, the passenger door opened and a little black dog ran out. A woman followed, chasing the dog down the sidewalk, shouting at the dog. We stopped taping. She scooped up the dog and scolded it as she carried it back to the van. Then she returned and took one look at me.

I immediately thought of my childhood bully. "No, it can't be!" I said to myself.

"I went to school with your sister…or, maybe, you! What's your name?" she demanded.

I shuddered. *The bully's back!* "Brenda," I immediately replied. *It is twenty-seven years later, and I am still conditioned to reply immediately.*

Before I could think of how to ask my question, she threw out the next question, "How old are you?"

"Thirty-seven."

"Then I went to school with you!"

Uh-ohhhh, could this be? Nahhh, no way! I try to keep my composure and all the while wanting to doubt my instinct. I reply, as nonchalantly as I can, "Oh, really…and what's your name?" *Please don't say it, pleeeeessseee!*

She says her name. *It's her! I can't believe it. Not the same one who beat up on me at Hayes Elementary School—and actually made me cry. No, not her. After twenty-seven years, could it really be her?* Once again, I try hard to control my emotions. I say her name, pause and then repeat it. I feign thought…"Are you the [her name] who used to beat up on me at Hayes?"

"Yes, I was," she replied sheepishly.

"Wow!" What else could I say?

She briefly explained that she did not have a proper upbringing and beating up others was the way she coped. *Yeah, beating up on ME!* She assured me that she had changed. *I should hope so!. She has kids of her own now.*

"Wow!" I said again. *I couldn't think of anything else to say. After all these years, I had come face-to-face with the bully, at my father's estate sale.*

I was kind to her as she walked though the house. In fact, as she was walking around looking at things to buy, I introduced her to a few other people as the girl who used to beat up on me in grade school. Embarrassed, she tried to silence me by furling her brows and shaking her head while she placed her index finger over her lips. *With newly gained confidence that came from her weakness, I continued flaunting the truth.*

Ironically, I was thrilled and thankful that she introduced herself. I was able to close that one area of my life. Many years of therapy were prevented in just a few minutes during my father's estate sale.

Our meeting had a funny ending. She approached the estate sale administrator with her purchases. I introduced her to the administrator as a person with whom I had went to grade school. This was all I said. The administrator looked at the items and totaled what she owed. After she paid and left, the people I had earlier told the truth to, and who were waiting to pay for their items, asked if I tried pulling her hair or even kicking her out of the house. The administrator looked puzzled. They explained that she used to beat up on me. The administrator looked at me and said, "I didn't know she used to beat up on you. I gave her a discount!"

᠅　᠅

FOLLOW FIVE PACES BEHIND.

One day in support group, one of the participants asked if it was normal for her mother to follow a few paces back instead of walking by her side. I smiled. I had the same question.

While in Taiwan, I noticed how families walked *together*. The eldest male walks in front of his wife and children, who follow a few paces behind. In Taipei, the capital of Taiwan, I especially noticed this with older men. It looked unusual when compared to our western culture. Chivalry suggests that a gentleman walk beside a lady, open the door for her, and then follow her through the door.

Mardig was chivalrous. In Milwaukee, when we walked together and approached a door, he'd hold it open and then follow me inside. But a few months after moving him to California, we noticed that when David and I went out with him he'd always follow a few steps behind us. Or, if I took him shopping, he'd say, "You go ahead, I'm coming." If I slowed down, he'd slow down. It was almost as if an invisible barrier existed between us that kept us a certain distance apart.

We thought this was strange. Sometimes we felt as if a little puppy dog was trailing behind us. Other times, we felt he was throwing a temper tantrum and wanted to follow at a distance.

During the support group another possibility was raised. People with Alzheimer's followed because they felt safer being able to see their caregivers in front of them.

Nonetheless, it posed some problems when Mardig would get distracted and walk somewhere else, and we'd have to retrace our steps to find him.

∿   ∿

BREAKING THE LAW...
One particularly windy day, Lew, Mardig, and I went to the California Poppy Preserve in the Antelope Valley. We took plenty of pictures and videotaped my father committing a crime.

The orange-red poppy is California's state flower. From what we've been told, picking a California poppy is against the law. My father didn't know. He bent down, saw the pretty flower, and plucked it right out of the ground! He carried his victorious acquisition with pride. Fortunately, he didn't get caught.

∿   ∿

THERE ARE NO GOOD-BYES—ONLY HELLOS.

Good-byes are difficult. When you care about someone, you wish there were no good-byes. Lovers have a hard time saying good-bye when ending their telephone conversations. "No, you say it!"

"No, you say it and then we'll hang up."

"I don't want to hang up."

"Okay, we won't say good-bye."

They go back and forth for five, ten, sometimes fifteen minutes, because lovers don't want to say, good-bye.

It's no different when your loved one has Alzheimer's. David and I have learned that there are no good-byes, only hellos.

Each time we visit Mardig, we greet him with a hearty "Hello!"

He furls his brow, looks at our faces, and then he gives us a big smile. "Boy, am I glad to see both of you!" he usually exclaims.

After we've spent an hour or two with him and we're ready to leave, we usually just walk away. Sometimes, he'll say, "You're free to stay here and do what you want. I need to…" and he'll walk away, or he'll sit down and rest. Whatever he does, we watch him for a while. When he enters the world he creates in his mind, we see he has forgotten us and we leave.

It seemed cruel at first to walk away from him like that. But he really does not remember. When we said, "Good-bye" it was more painful for him.

"When am I going to see you again?" he'd ask. Or, "Where are you going?" Or, "I'll come with you."

We've learned that if we simply let him be, there is no need to say good-bye.

This has had a profound effect on us as well. We realize that one day, he will no longer be with us. So, we treasure each moment, knowing that each visit may be our last.

Chapter 17

TIME WITH OTHERS

SOMETIMES MY THOUGHTS TAKE ME BACK TO THE DAYS WHEN MY father first came to live with us. It was the fall of 1996, a season filled with lots of social opportunities. I enjoyed seeing Mardig smile and laugh with my friends and business partners. He showered every other day and was always nicely dressed. We even took his clothes to the cleaners. He would comment on the creases in his pants. He looked sharp, he was polite, and people enjoyed spending time with him. After all, he was the consummate gentleman.

$\backsim$ $\backsim$

MARDIG ATTENDS OUR BUSINESS MEETINGS.
Because Mardig wandered, we had to keep an eye on him. David and I began to take turns staying home to watch Mardig; however, over the weeks, we realized this was limiting the progress we made building our business. Both of us needed to be present at some meetings, and so, one evening, we brought Mardig along. Initially we felt uncomfortable. After all, how many people bring their parent to a business meeting, much less one who has Alzheimer's and occasionally says and does things that are embarrassing?

Our fears were unfounded. Mardig turned out to be a joy for our business partners. He received a lot of attention and provided enough distraction to balance the seriousness of our intense planning sessions. He admitted he was getting *spoiled* with all the attention. Our business partners genuinely enjoyed him and wanted Mardig to come to future meetings.

If I had any concerns about our partners just trying to be polite, my concerns evaporated. The following example illustrates the kind of attention Mardig received.

One of our business partners, a petite young lady with long black hair, immediately took a liking to him. She smiled, laughed at his jokes, and gave him back and shoulder massages. Before one of our meetings, she invited Mardig to the swing set in the backyard of our host's house. Watching them swing like children, smiling and giggling, I knew I had to buy a videocamera.

I have since captured many special moments of my father. Such sweet memories.

↝   ↝

SPECIAL FRIENDS HELP CARE FOR MARDIG.

Less than one month after Mardig arrived in California, I had to take a business trip. Having arranged his participation in the Adult Day Care Center, the only thing we had to coordinate was his care in the early mornings and early evenings. Mardig participated at the Adult Day Care Center for six-hours each day. David was gone for thirteen hours—a four-hour commute, plus his nine-hour workday. What would Mardig do during the remaining seven hours?

Lots of planning and ingenuity, not to mention heavy reliance on my father's charm, helped us make arrangements for his care by two very special friends. First, we had to be certain our plans would work. Jan would take care of Mardig in the mornings, and Sally would care for him in the evenings.

Sally was already caring for her father so we felt assured she could manage Mardig. Besides, Sally's husband, Ken, was there to help if necessary. Also, their home was fully encircled by a fence with a locked wrought iron entryway. Mardig would not be able to wander too far if he felt the urge.

Jan was in an entirely different situation. She would be the sole caregiver for Mardig after her husband left for work at 6:15 a.m. She lived on a quarter-acre in a rural area accessed by a busy street close to her home. We decided to do a trial run with Jan before I left on my trip.

At 4:30 a.m. David took Mardig to Dave's and Jan's house where he would stay for three to four hours until Jan took him to adult day care. This worked out nicely. Jan told us they'd spend their early mornings reading the paper, drinking juice, or sharing a breakfast muffin. He repeatedly asked for maps wanting to know where he was, she said.

It is sad to realize that my father didn't know where he was. Everything looked so different in the high desert—a large valley surrounded by mountains which still offer a 360° view of the horizon; a valley dotted with Joshua trees which have given way to new housing developments. In this strange and unfamiliar place, my father drew comfort from kind and loving people. Yet, he never realized he achieved his and my mother's long-held dream to move to California.

Our plan worked. This would be the routine while I was away. It was fortunate that Jan and Mardig genuinely admired one another. He enjoyed her immensely and began calling her "the barefoot lady." Jan loved to go barefoot and rarely wore shoes or socks at home. Mardig had poor recall of names. (I have this weakness too.) Whenever we talked about Jan, we'd refer to her as "the barefoot lady." He easily remembered this nickname and could describe what she looked like and on what side of town she lived.

Jan enjoyed Mardig because he was pleasant and because he reminded her of her father. One day, David and I brought Mardig to visit Jan and Dave. It was a cool fall afternoon, and David, Dave, and my father went out into the backyard to look at Dave's progress on restoring his collection of old Corvettes. Jan and I stood in the kitchen, where it was warmer, and looked out the window while sipping our drinks. Suddenly, Jan grabbed my forearm. Hardly able to contain herself, she exclaimed, "Just look at him!" She pointed toward Mardig. "He looks so much like my father!"

Even one of Jan's newer neighbors, our former business partner and a good friend, recognized the special relationship Jan and Mardig shared. She sent me the following e-mail while I was in Mississippi.

> Hey Girl!
> Sounds like you are having a really good time....
> We are planning a show on Friday...When you get back we need to toss over some ideas...
> I saw Jan one morning with your father. She was showing him the mailbox. She must be a wonderful woman. I hope to get to know her better.
> Have a good trip in the South. That's my old stomping grounds and I miss it much.
> See you on your return.

Sometimes gifts can be given (Mardig reminding Jan of her father) even in a time of one's own need (I needed someone to care for Mardig during my absence).

At the end of each day, Sally picked up Mardig from the Adult Day Care Center. Two or three days a week, Sally's father also attended day care, so it was convenient for her to pick up both of them. But every other day, when her father stayed at home, she made a special trip to bring Mardig to her house. He read, watched TV, or looked at maps until David came two or three hours later. Sometimes, when David was late (Los Angeles traffic is unpredictable), Mardig would join Sally and her family for dinner.

Wow! Aren't friends truly valuable?

◡   ∾

MARDIG GOES TO LAS VEGAS.
We decided to take Mardig to Las Vegas during Thanksgiving. David's parents live there, and his brother, Bruce, would be visiting. We could be together, enjoy Thanksgiving dinner, and then visit the casinos. We didn't know how Mardig would fare, but we packed an overnight bag for him with extras and decided to head out early Thanksgiving morning. I sat in the backseat with the videocamera and Mardig sat in the front with David.

The four-hour drive to Las Vegas was relatively uneventful. David and Mardig talked. I napped and occasionally shot some footage, especially when we got into town. Mardig was surprised we were in Las Vegas. Despite his awareness of what city he was in, I don't think he realized we drove from California. I believe he thought we made the four-hour trip by car from Milwaukee.

Once we arrived near David's parents' home, we stopped at a grocery store to pick up some goodies. Then we went to their house. I stood back with the videocamera, hoping to catch the moment the door opened and David's parents would see my father. I doubt Mardig knew who we were visiting. David's mother greeted my father first with a big smile and an awkward hug. None of us knew what to expect. It didn't take long, however, for all of us to settle in and feel at home while enjoying one another's company.

Mardig read, watched a little television with Bruce, and enjoyed the hearty Thanksgiving meal amidst all the conversation and laughter. Bruce would take the videocamera and zoom in really close without us realizing. We laughed when we saw the funny close-ups of us chewing our food, gesturing, or talking.

That night, Mardig slept in the guest room and we slept on the floor in the living room. Because he wandered, we needed to be watchful. We didn't sleep well that night. He got up in the middle of the night and was confused. He wanted to use the bathroom and didn't remember where it was. David helped him find the bathroom and then explained where he was. After David's cajoling, Mardig went back to bed. *Oh, the sacrifices "parents" make.*

We spent part of the following afternoon at Caesar's Palace. David's father taught Mardig how to play the slots. We watched as my father seemed to enjoy himself amidst the noise and flashing lights. He even won a few quarters! We took him to the IMAX feature on whales. He enjoyed it, despite feeling a little seasick. We then went to a pub, and he ordered fish and chips. Afterward, David and I took him to a candy store. He enjoyed that the most!

It was late afternoon and there was a four-hour drive ahead of us. We hugged David's parents, said our good-byes, and left Caesar's Palace to drive home. Mardig seemed fine. After sunset, we stopped for gas and I used the rest room. This stop at the gas station really confused Mardig. He wanted to go back. He insisted we were heading in the wrong direction. *He was so convincing, we questioned whether we had made a wrong turn.* Mardig wanted to go back...to Milwaukee. We struggled to help him understand. Eventually, he cooperated, but unconvincingly.

We hoped that once we arrived home, he would see his things and be comforted by familiar surroundings. But we were not so fortunate. Mardig thought we were tricking him by reproducing his room and things in this *new* place. He insisted he had to go home, that people were expecting him, and that he would visit this place later. It took us a couple hours to get him to change into his pajamas and go to bed. He didn't understand, but was too tired to insist any longer.

The following morning, he was fine and as cheerful as ever.

⌁   ∾

MARDIG FLIES TO CATALINA ISLAND.
My father had been living in the skilled nursing facility for one and a half months when the opportunity arose for him to visit Catalina Island. He had so many dreams of travel. We wanted to provide him this opportunity before he became too incapacitated to go out. As it turned out, this was to be his final outing.

In March 1997, our good friend, Lew, was planning a trip to Catalina Island. A superb still photographer, Lew wanted to visit the island to take pictures.

He had a fine rapport with my father. Mardig couldn't explain why he felt close to Lew, having only met him a few months earlier. Nonetheless, we thought this would be a fine opportunity for the *two buddies* to share a fun adventure.

David and I had flown to Catalina a year earlier, and thought Mardig would enjoy the trip. We proposed the idea to Lew. At sixty, Lew's age falsely represented the youthful vigor with which he lived life. Before he replied, we threw in an enticement. The ferry would take an hour. I proposed that if he agreed to take Mardig, we would pick up the tab for the fifteen-minute helicopter flight to the island.

He agreed.

All we had to do was coordinate the logistics. We made arrangements with the nursing facility to have Mardig dressed and ready at 5:00 a.m. We wrote a letter giving Lew permission to care for my father and to make any decisions for him should the need arise. We also gave Lew Mardig's identification. David gave Lew a cell phone, and I gave him our videocamera.

We agreed to meet Lew at the skilled nursing facility at 4:30 a.m. We were surprised to see Mardig was fully dressed and ready to go. We signed him out, and he accompanied us outside. A colorful array of orange, pink, and brown introduced the March sun's arrival. Lew took a few pictures, one with the multi-colored palette as a backdrop. We wished both of them well, exchanged hugs. Then David and I watched Lew and Mardig drive away. It was like seeing our child head off to camp. We didn't know what to expect and felt a little nervous, but we hoped for the best. They would drive down to the port in Long Beach to board a helicopter—my father's first flight in one.

Days later, Lew wrote a detailed diary of their journey and had two sets made of all the pictures he took featuring my father and the Casino, the Wrigley Museum and grounds, various flora, and the glass-bottom boat tour. He made this special for us by giving us the photos, a photo album, and colorful stationery of seashells and images of the sea. In the end, we assembled a beautiful keepsake of my father's journey to Catalina Island.

Chapter 18

WHAT IS THE MEANING OF LIFE?

I don't believe this book would be complete without considering the answer to one question. One afternoon while sitting in the facility's activity room, with Mardig sleeping in the chair by my side, I looked at the residents and occasionally glanced at the talk show on TV. I thought about what it would be like to live in an Alzheimer's skilled nursing facility some day. I just couldn't stop wondering, "What is the meaning of life?"

IS IT WEARING SOMEONE ELSE'S CLOTHES?

Residents' families learn to get used to a variety of things. One is that residents will wear each other's clothes. David and I try to overlook instances when Mardig wears other people's clothes or others wear his. We try to focus on the more important issues of his care. For example, before he went into the facility, we arranged to have his eyes examined and bought him a very nice pair of glasses—$250 for a pair with light-weight plastic lenses that would not push too hard on the bridge of his nose. We even bought a bright red strap to hold his glasses around his neck when he was not using them.

He lost both. We told the social services representative, and she found them. He lost them again. They were found. He lost them again. This went on for two or three months, after which they were never found. We were told Mardig left his glasses in other resident's rooms and took the glasses he found in those rooms. We soon learned that he had an affinity for women's glasses with large colorful frames. For a two-month period, he'd have on a different pair when we visited him. Actually, they looked rather nice on him.

David and I learned it doesn't matter whose clothes you wear, just as long as they are clean, they fit, they are comfortable, and you are happy wearing them.

∻   ∻

Is it watching the Oprah Winfrey show?

I was seated next to my father in the activity room one afternoon when he drifted off to sleep shortly after sitting down. Being one who must have something to do every minute of every day, I started feeling antsy at not having my work with me. I tried to watch TV, but my mind raced with all the things I had to do. Then again, Oprah Winfrey had a special show where she and her guest, Tina Turner, were making people's dreams come true. I admire both of these women and watched a little as I tried to calm my mind. The thought occurred to me to leave. *I couldn't sneak out and leave my father there!* (This was before I realized that there are no good-byes.) If he was tired enough to fall asleep in his chair, I wanted him to rest. So I waited until he awoke.

I sat there and looked around at the other residents. One woman sat in a wheelchair, crying out and pounding on the tray table. Her face expressed dire urgency and great pain. The image of a mother screaming in emotional agony at the loss of her husband and/or son in a war-torn region came into my mind. I wanted to reach out to this woman, to comfort her, yet I could not. *What if she needed my attention for a long time and Mardig woke up? Could I tear myself away from her to be with him again?*

I continued looking around the room. An older, overweight man wearing a baseball cap, who I usually saw walking along the hallway near Mardig's room, sat, staring. Whenever I walked near him, I was on guard as I never knew what to expect. His mouth was slightly open and saliva dripped down onto his shirt. His eyes were deep and intense-looking, and I feared one day he'd lunge out at me and start screaming. Then there was Elizabeth. She was carefully turning the pages of a magazine. Starting at the top of each page, I watched her head slowly move down as she scanned the page, top to bottom, before turning to the next one. She had a look of peacefulness about her.

Elizabeth and Jonathan, her husband, spent most of their lives helping others. They are in their early eighties. Elizabeth was diagnosed with Alzheimer's a few years earlier. It saddened me to see her. She was an author and a teacher. For years, many considered her a source of knowledge and wisdom.

I had only recently met them when Jonathan, who attends the same support group I do, was kind enough to share her book with me. I read most of *The Living Atoms and You,* and then met with Jonathan to ask him a few questions. Elizabeth had written about the significant role atoms play in our everyday lives—physically, spiritually, mentally, and emotionally.

Why? Why was Elizabeth destined to live the rest of her days here in this facility with Alzheimer's? Why was the woman pounding on her tray table? Why was that man left to live his remaining days drooling and with Alzheimer's? Why was my father enduring this disease?

I was struck deeply by the residents I observed. On the television, I saw Oprah give a woman $58,000 to pay off all her debts. During one moment, I witnessed a person's dream come true. I switched my attention between Oprah and the residents. During another moment, I noticed residents oblivious of the TV. Oprah making this woman's dream come true didn't matter. The commercial break didn't matter. These people didn't care whether they had money or not, whether they had a more flavorful cup of coffee or not, whether they had a new car or not. None of these things mattered.

What mattered to them? I cannot imagine. But Oprah, Tina Turner, the woman whose dreams just came true celebrating joyously...none of this mattered to the people in this activity room.

↙ ∾

So, what matters? What is the meaning of life?
While sitting in the activity room that afternoon, I was profoundly moved. So many of us, comparatively healthy, are driven by our needs, goals, wants, aspirations. We need to be successful in life. What does

this mean? If we were to judge what successful meant by watching television, we'd say it was having lots of money. Don't we need money to buy a new car every two years? Don't we need money to eat at the finest restaurants? Don't we need money to buy exquisite gold jewelry accented with real diamonds? (After all, isn't a man's love measured by the percent of his yearly salary he spends on a diamond?) *Do these things really matter?*

Well, I suppose it depends on each person's perspective.

Over the years, especially since the Northridge earthquake, I have been disposing of the unnecessary things in my life. Because I live in California, I have taken a catastrophic view of living. *What if the big one (earthquake) hits? What is the absolute essential stuff I would take with me?* This forces me to keep only what is necessary (with a few extras). Anything more may cause me to be indecisive at a critical moment and to lose those things that are important to me (if I can save even those). Consequently, I do not collect knickknacks (too much maintenance to keep them clean, watch over them, etc.). I give away clothes I do not wear. I do not accept or take things I cannot use.

The residents in this Alzheimer's facility helped me get a perspective on what life may *really* be about. *I'm only thirty-eight. There's a lot I have not experienced yet. Two years ago, I had no idea what I would learn about this disease.*

What I do see is that the residents do not own a lot of things. In fact, there were humorous sayings among some of the residents' families, "Everything that enters the facility is shared by all." "Socialism is alive and well in here." Rarely does anyone wear jewelry. Most don't have a wallet or purse, and they do not carry money. Most of them wear cotton-polyester blend sweat shirts and pants, which are comfortable and serve multiple purposes (for walking and sleeping). They bathe every other day. They sleep in simple beds, with white polyester-cotton blend sheets, and cotton blankets. They eat three meals a day that are custom-prepared for them based on their nutritional needs.

Occasionally they complain about wanting to go somewhere or needing something. Overall, they seem to be peaceful, occupied with their own thoughts and the worlds they create for themselves. They are like children who occupy themselves for hours with their imaginations. Their disease helps them believe that they travel to many places. In recent months my father's been to England, Africa, Wisconsin, Illinois, Boston, and New York. Many drive every day. Mardig took the car to visit Ma. Some take the bus. All see their families at one time or another; especially their parents. This is how they survive. And they've made me think about what's really important in our lives— memories of fun times with other people.

Life is the process of creating special memories with people. These are life's real treasures when we have nothing more.

I smile at this realization. After all, we never know if we've lived life right until we're done. Then it's too late. So I try to observe others' decisions and the impact their decisions have upon their lives. It's easier to look at someone else's life to better learn about our own. This is why I watch A&E's *Biography*. I wonder what in these residents' lives leaves some with great pain (e.g., the woman who was pounding on her tray table), others with warm memories, and the rest at peace (e.g., Elizabeth). Is this even reasonable to wonder? Why is it some people get visitors and others do not?

I contrast my thoughts to the images portrayed in today's advertisements. What's it all for? In the end, what does it matter that I drove a convertible along the entire California coastline? What does it matter that I had dinner at a five-star restaurant in Washington, D.C.? What does it matter that I receive annual invitations from the Governor to a barbecue before the Kentucky Derby? What does it matter that I earned 1000-plus percent annualized interest on a few of my stocks and options investments? What does it matter that I had front-row center seats at *Phantom of the Opera*?

Will any of these things matter while I'm pounding my fist on the tray table attached to my chair, scanning each page of an old magazine, drooling on my shirt, or sleeping in my chair in front of the television set in an Alzheimer's facility's activity room?

Chapter 19

LITTLE THINGS
MATTER THE MOST

 *W*HEN I AM WITH MY FATHER, I FOCUS ON THE PRESENT. I remind myself to accept him as he *is,* not as he was or could be. As the disease progresses and takes its toll on his brain this becomes more difficult. I find it challenging to watch him struggle to make sense of his surroundings. I find it increasingly difficult emotionally to listen as Mardig desperately tries to make sense of his world, as his vocabulary slowly escapes him, and as he struggles to find the words to express himself. I watch him try to recall his family—his children, his wife, his brothers, etc. His world is slowly shrinking, and he is left only with the little things, his memories of *mere* incidents from years gone by.

In the hours I've spent with Mardig, I've learned it's the little things that matter most, not the big things. When I look back upon my life, it's the little things I vividly recall. When I weave these little things together, a very pleasant sensation comes over me, and I rest back in my chair and sigh with a smile.

⌁   ⌁

MARDIG'S 87TH BIRTHDAY
David and I wanted to bring Mardig home to celebrate his birthday, but this was impractical. He considers the nursing facility where he lives to be his home, and he feels uncomfortable when he leaves its

security. We don't understand this, because we think a change of pace would be nice. *After all, wouldn't he like to go out for a little while?*

We made arrangements to bring the birthday celebration to him. We ordered a butter-cream frosted marble cake. The sweeter the better. He loves sweets! We ordered it to be decorated with confetti, ribbons, his name, and "Happy 87th Birthday!" These days, he does not recall how old he is—usually he thinks he is in his thirties or fifties. We bought noise makers and a cake knife (actually, a long-serrated bread knife), plastic forks, and paper plates.

We invited people who helped care for him while he was living with us—Sally, Jan, Dave, and Roberta. We invited Jonathan and his wife, Elizabeth, and the staff from the facility. We wanted a little crowd to celebrate Mardig's achievement—eighty-seven years on this challenging journey called life.

On his birthday (it was mine too!) we had a little gathering, just as I'd envisioned. Mardig was happy and even a bit alarmed at all the fuss for him. We still aren't sure he knew it was his birthday. And for a moment...when he picked up the long-serrated knife to cut the cake...

Mardig cut a piece off the corner of the cake—a very heavily frosted piece. He then carefully balanced this sweet morsel on the end of the long knife blade. We watched closely, wanting to grab the knife out of his hand, and yet frozen still with fear that we might startle him. *I definitely had to give my father credit. He took great pains to be careful.* Still, he did have Alzheimer's. Carefully balancing the cake on the knife, he slowly turned it toward his mouth. We watched, totally speechless. Then someone gasped. It was the activity director. Mardig looked up and pulled the knife out of his mouth. He was unharmed. We broke out laughing with relief and rushed to him with a plastic fork. Then we sang "Happy Birthday" as Mardig continued to eat his cake. He had a big smile, with frosting on the outside of his mouth. He was having fun, and so were we.

What a birthday! Even though it was my birthday too, Mardig stole the show with the knife incident.

⌐   ∿

MY MOTHER IRONING

I remember my mother spending a lot of time each week ironing. I remember her ironing upstairs in the master bedroom of our home. I remember warm summer days when she'd iron downstairs in the living room or the sunroom. When the weather was especially nice—a warm gentle breeze blowing, she would take the ironing outdoors. She'd iron outside of the sunroom, near the dining room windows. At first I felt funny watching her iron outdoors. *People are not supposed to iron outdoors!* I would stay inside because I was embarrassed and I didn't want to be seen by the neighbors. Eventually, I grew used to watching her and even volunteered to help her carry clothes and the iron outside.

I remember her ironing my father's work clothes—pants, shirts (both dress and work), handkerchiefs and even boxer shorts. I'd stand by her in the living room and watch, sometimes trying to help, but mostly getting in her way. She would put the ironed clothes on the floor, and I'd play with the neatly arranged pants and shirts. I'd fold the legs on my father's pants every which way to see what kind of funny contortions I could create. I'd do the same with the arms of his shirts. She'd shoosh me away, but I'd come back.

I used to wonder, "Will I have to iron so much when I grow up? It takes so much time! It never ends! I'm not going to do this when I grow up. But, *who* will? Maybe I'll hire someone to do it for me."

When my parents rented our bedrooms to others, before my sister and I were born, my mother used to do the cleaning and ironing. She would iron linen sheets and pillowcases.

So I ironed. I decided to iron the few things of hers I brought back from Milwaukee. Her embroidery ("tsera khordz" she would say in Armenian, which literally means handiwork) lay on the ironing board as I decided how to carefully iron these treasures without harming them. I stood in our guest room and ironed. I ironed doilies, handkerchiefs, pillowcases, tablecloths, etc. All of these featured her *tsera khordz*. I stood ironing. My already weak wrist was beginning to ache.

It's been over thirty years since I thought about Ma ironing, and now I was reliving the past. Except, I *became* her for a moment, while

I envisioned "little Brenda" standing to my right by *her* side. I stood there peacefully ironing, watching me *(her)* from my young self's vantage point, wanting to help. I carefully laid out the material and then glided the iron over it, being careful not to accidentally press a crease into the material or get the tip of the iron caught in her embroidered designs. *Wow, such work! Such labor-intensive work.*

There I was, wearing my little wrinkled dress, white anklets with embroidered designs, and black patent leather shoes. I wanted to help my mother finish her ironing.

And here I was the adult who did not want to spend the weekend ironing. (David and I take our clothes to the laundry.) Still I had a need to iron these things. I felt I was honoring my mother. It was the one time I felt I was able to understand the extent of her responsibility. She would say, "Wait until you have kids, you'll understand." Well, David and I are both in our late thirties and we still have not started a family. *But at this moment, I think I understand. If only a little.*

In honor of and in the memory of my mother, I felt renewed strength. I stood and ironed. I ironed all of the pieces of her *tsera khordz*, wrapped them carefully in tissue paper and placed them inside white gift boxes. I will pull them out from time to time and display them on my furniture. I will *use* them. Ma had packed them away. Each time I look at them or a guest comments on them, I will acknowledge my mother's efforts. In this way, her work will be seen and she will be remembered.

✦   ~

SIBLING RIVALRY

There are three of us. My brother is eight years older than me. My sister is the middle child and older than me by two years. The more I think about our upbringing, the more I realize we were raised to be competitive.

If there's anything that fostered healthy competition, it was when we played checkers with Mardig. Of course, Ma occasionally added some unfair competitive advantage when she sat close enough to Mardig to sneak one of his pieces *off* the checker board! She could do this quite easily since he focused intensely on each move and seemed to lack peripheral vision. Most often, we kids would laugh, because we couldn't believe Mardig actually focused so hard. This would lead to his puzzled look and our confession of the dirty deed. Ma, having been caught, would look off in another direction with pristine innocence. *Moi?*

Our height was another source of competition. My brother was the tallest, then my sister, and then little ol' me! I still have not won this sibling competition. But I finally grew taller than my father! That was a major coup.

So there I was, wondering what I could win because my older sister and brother were so much better at everything than me. (They made certain I remembered how much better they were, too.)

When I think of it, it's truly amazing how differently kids grow into adults. When my friends and I discuss how our upbringings have affected us I realize I could have turned out really different. I could have just given up. Or, I could have sought highly competitive situations where winning was the only thing that mattered.

Still, what could I do to win? What was the one thing I could be better at than my sister or brother? If they are older and always had a head start, what was left?

The time came when I graduated from high school at the age of sixteen. I was in my second year of college and did not like living with my parents. I was the rebel, the one who tried new things, the one who often went contrary to our parents' wishes. I was the independent, know-it-all eighteen-year old. I needed to spread my wings. I moved out a few months after my eighteenth birthday. This was a first! My sister moved out permanently soon after. She was twenty. My brother stayed at home until shortly before I arranged to sell Mardig's house. *He lost. He stayed at home until he was forty-six. I won! Ahhh, that's one victory for me!*

I believe I won in other areas as well. Unlike my siblings, without my parents' financial support I earned a college degree and went on to earn a graduate degree. It was very hard and the money would have been nice, but I learned a lot about survival and succeeding, despite many obstacles and temptations along the way. Afterwards, it was no longer important to *win*. I proved to myself I could set goals and achieve them. I did not need to compare myself to my brother or sister. What was important were the goals I accomplished—for me.

Chapter 20

A RARE GIFT INDEED

O NE FALL AFTERNOON, THE WIND GUSTS WERE SO POWERFUL I had difficulty keeping my car in the lane on the freeway. I had just received very encouraging comments from the other authors at our monthly North Los Angeles County Women Writers' Network luncheons. My thoughts were focused on this book while my car swerved with the forces of the wind.

I was going to visit Mardig. A few pages of this book were careful-ly laid out on the passenger seat. I had selected them based on their interest to my father. I couldn't wait to sit by his side as he read my tribute to him.

What a rare gift indeed. My father is alive as I complete this book. I wanted him to read at least a portion of it, even though his concen-tration is not what it used to be. He could no longer make much sense of what he read. What he derived meaning from sometimes became his reality. Months earlier, he retrieved an old issue of *National Geographic* and read an article about poachers in Africa. He spent the rest of the day thinking he was living in Africa trying to stop the poachers. He'd sometimes invite us to join him on these missions. Another time, he had to leave immediately and go to England, his imagined homeland, to fight in the war (World War II). Realizing this, I was prepared to accept whatever he would do—whether he chose to read this, ignore it, whatever.

So often when we accomplish something in life, we think of our parents and wonder what they would say. Some are fortunate in that they can still call their parents, visit them, or invite them to visit. They can still share their achievements. Others' parents are no longer living or in such poor health, they cannot share the joys of their children's achievements. Perhaps the desire for our parents' praise lives long into our adulthood. Aren't we still yearning for a warm smile, a compliment, a pat on the back or hug, that only a parent can give?

～   ～

I FOUND MARDIG WALKING IN THE HALLWAY. He looked up at me, stared deeply, and then broke into a big smile after I greeted him with a hearty "Hello, Mardig!" He started talking about a few things, but I could not make sense of what he was saying. Alzheimer's seems to have progressed quickly for him. Still, I always listen to him, with a warm smile and a lot of nods and yeses. I paraphrase some of the things he says, even though they don't make sense. This makes him feel comfortable about being able to communicate his thoughts.

We walked in the hallways and talked awhile. I told him I had a surprise for him. He smiled, as anyone would in anticipation of a surprise. We looked for a place to sit. A large empty recreation room provided a nice quiet place to settle down. We sat, side by side at a table, Mardig to my right.

I pulled out the cover page of the book and handed it to him. He began reading. I thought he would make the connection between *a tribute to my father* and the author's name, his daughter. He didn't say a word. Still, I knew if he understood what he was reading, he would be proud—very proud. He would be happy "one of his own," as he used to say, "had made something of *him*self." (He typically referred to me as a *he*.)

He held his hand out for the next page. I handed him the introduction. As he read this page, a few residents came in.

They walked around us, and a woman sat to my left. I looked at her and smiled, she smiled back. She was holding a little stuffed white bunny in her left hand while adoringly petting its head with her right. I thought about my sister and her two bunnies.

Mardig continued reading. After awhile, I asked, "So, what do you think?"

"Nice history," he replied. He resumed reading.

After a few minutes, it appeared that he was reading and rereading only the bottom part of this introductory page.

I asked if he had any questions.

I was surprised at his response: "I'm amazed at the amount of money *he* acquired and that *he* changed from his home to the family home."

Wow, this was about him and yet he thought he was reading about someone else! He had read about the $100,000 accumulated from his GE stock and about moving from his home to our home.

Just then another resident walked to where we were seated and stood inches from his right elbow. Mardig looked at me, suggested that we put these materials away, and look at them later. He spoke in Armenian.

It was hard getting used to the lack of privacy in the skilled nursing facility. Then again, I had no choice because it happened so frequently. How do you ask someone with Alzheimer's to go elsewhere? Each resident needs a lot of nods and gentleness. I've come to realize that even though they look over our shoulders, they really don't know what they are seeing. Occasionally, the staff and aides saw this and gently cajoled a resident away to give my father and me privacy.

I encouraged Mardig to continue reading and alerted him that the person by his side had just left. I then handed him the first page of the chapter, "Little Things Matter the Most." Pointing to the section describing his 87th birthday, I told him, "Mardig, this is about *your* 87th birthday party, which was held *here!*" He started reading.

The thought then occurred to me that this was a *rare gift, indeed.* Here I am writing a tribute to him, and he is reading it! Why not include his remarks? I took the pages he had already read and, on the back sides, which were blank, started writing notes before I forgot the details. I noted how we walked the hallways and talked, what his initial reactions were to the introduction of this book, and his other comments.

When he spoke about what he was reading, he used the third person, saying, "he." After a few minutes, I asked him if he knew whose 87th birthday this was. He replied, "The two of us, I guess." He quietly read for a while longer and then spoke in the third person, saying "he" and "him."

I clarified his response with, "Mardig, this is about you." I'm not sure he agreed.

He continued reading the section about my mother ironing. Again, I asked who he was reading about. "Pop," he replied, "since it's downstairs. Ma would be upstairs," he added. *Was he recalling people based on where they were in the house?*

"Do you remember this?" I asked, wondering if he remembered my mother ironing.

"Yeah, playing with Pa's clothes—putting 'em in shape." *It was us if he was I!* Then he asked, "What are they doing now?"

He continued to read and sometimes made comments. I watched him most of the time. My attention was occasionally drawn to the room we were in. A woman sat in a "gerichair"—a type of wheelchair that restrains residents who are too agitated, so they don't injure themselves. She was wheeled into the room by one of the aides and positioned toward our right side. She had short curly white hair. I noticed she was wearing a T-shirt proclaiming something funny. She had a pale pink sheet upon her lap. She took great care to fold it and then unfold it, making certain the sides and ends came together. She repeated this action a half-dozen times while I watched her. She was totally immersed in her work, never noticing me looking at her for a few minutes while my father read.

Mardig spoke, and my attention shifted back to him. "...unrelated situation sparking warm memories..." is all I heard. Then he pointed with his right index finger to each word as he read a few lines aloud. "My mother ironing...I remember my mother spending a lot of time each week ironing. I remember her ironing upstairs in the master bedroom of our home. I remember some warm summer days when she'd iron downstairs in the living room or the sunroom." He continued reading quietly.

194 ~ "WHERE'S MY SHOES?"

After he read awhile he reached the portion about when we'd play checkers and my mother would take his pieces. I asked him if he knew who this was about. "I'm getting to it," he replied then added, "Pop."

"Are *you* in here?" I asked, emphasizing "you."

"No."

"But you know these…"

"…situations. Yeah." he completed my sentence.

He stopped reading, looked outside, and then turned to me. "Things outside home…they been taken care of?" *Wow! He was aware of the windy day.*

"Yes," I replied. He looked into my eyes to be sure that I meant it. He was always concerned that things were taken care of.

He took another page and pointed to a paragraph. I looked at it. It was in the sibling rivalry section where I talked about our height being another source of competition. I asked him if he remembered who this was about. "About Pa because he was the earner," he answered.

Then he read a short paragraph aloud: "When I think of it, it's truly amazing how differently kids grow into adults…." When he finished, I said, "This is about your children, Mardig." There was no reply.

In the end, he stuck with it. He read the entire manuscript I brought for him to read—seven pages in all.

If I wanted recognition or appreciation, there was none to be given in the traditional sense. But if I, his daughter, wanted the rare and good fortune to have the opportunity to see my father read my tribute to him before he died, I GOT IT!

I reiterated: "Mardig, this is a book I am writing about *you*."

"It'll be interesting in years to come," he said.

Chapter 21

WHAT IF HE'S AWARE?

1 CAN'T STOP IT. The thought runs through my mind, "What if he's aware? What if my father knows what's really going on?"

Others have asked the same thing. "What if I sell my mother's home and later she becomes aware and insists on moving back?" one caregiver asks during support group. We laugh, because each of us has wondered this. Common sense may say otherwise, but it's still a concern.

David and I worked hard to get the home Mardig bought in 1952 ready to sell. My sister, brother, and I selected a few items of sentimental value and then I arranged to sell and/or donate the rest, depositing the proceeds in his estate.

Well, what if one day we're sitting together and talking, and Mardig straightens up and exclaims in very clear terms, "I'm finished here. I want to go home now."

Uh uhhh…hmmm, I don't know exactly how to tell you this, but nine months after we moved you to California, we sold your home in Milwaukee.

"You, *what?*" we imagine him asking. Except he would be more diplomatic. "Why would *you* sell *my* house?"

And then we would remain speechless, feeling utter embarrassment at what we had done.

Months earlier, he was aware. When he first moved to California with us, he was aware that he was forgetting. "I don't remember the

English language like I used to," he'd say. I'd encourage him to speak in Armenian. He would chuckle and add, "I'm forgetting. The words don't come as easily."

But now, what if he is truly aware? What if this was all an act? What if he's been studying how we will react?

Yes, I realize this seems farfetched, but I can't stop wondering.

Chapter 22

TREASURING SMALL MOMENTS

*I*T'S 5:50 P.M., TWENTY MINUTES INTO DINNERTIME when David and I visit Mardig at the skilled nursing facility. We walk into the lobby, and the receptionist greets us with a friendly "Hello." We ask to be let into the secured portion of the facility where the residents live. We hear the now-familiar *buzz* and turn the doorknob that electronically unlocks to let us in. We stand for a moment by the door surveying the place. Three halls extend in different directions; one directly ahead of us, another to our left, and the other to our right. We decide to walk ahead when one of the aides who speaks Armenian and spends time with my father informs us that Mardig is finishing his dinner in the dining room. She encourages us to join him.

Looking forward to a new experience, we walk toward the dining room. Residents' families are discouraged from visiting during meal times because, as it was once explained to us, the residents get distracted by new faces and get up without finishing their meals.

We hesitate at the doorway to the dining room, surveying the room and looking for Mardig. One of the activity coordinators, whose smile and attentions he greatly enjoys, approaches us and asks, "Are you looking for Martin?"

"Yes," we reply, pleased with the assistance.

"Come on in." She graciously motions for us to come in. "Come with me. He's back here eating his dinner," she explains.

We follow her to a row of tables toward the back where Mardig often likes to sit, especially since he is usually one of the last to show up for his meals. Residents who arrive earlier take the seats near the entrance.

"Marteen!" she exclaims, accentuating the "e"-sound. "Your daughter is here to see you!"

We thank her and she smiles and walks away to take care of another resident. Mardig looks up at me and then David. His eyes open wide.

"Oh, am I glad to see you!" he says, clasping his hands together. "Am I glad you came!" With this kind of an enthusiastic greeting, we decide to sit down. I sit next to him and David sits next to me.

"What did you come here for?" he asks.

"To see you!" we reply, with big smiles.

"Me?" he says, amazed that he is the reason for our visit.

"Yes, you!" I exclaim, kiddingly nudging his shoulder.

"Great!" he says and turns back to his meal.

He eats his meal and minds his own business. This is good. At least he is eating. David and I talk a little about our day. Another resident sitting across from Mardig gets our attention.

"Do you know where they parked my car?"

"Hmmm," I said, wondering how to respond. *We rarely know what a person is thinking.*

He adds, "Did they park it by LaSalle and Michigan?"

"LaSalle and Michigan, in Chicago?" I ask, hoping he will feel understood.

His eyes light up for an instant and then he nods.

"Yes," I say, "they parked it right where you asked them to."

"Good," he says. "Well, I'm going to go get it then."

I look at David and ask, "What is this? Is everyone from Chicago?"

My father lived in Chicago before moving to Milwaukee. Even in the nursing facility he often spoke of places he remembered in Chicago. One of his roommates in the facility was also from Chicago. He used to tell me stories of how Mardig (his imaginary brother) and he used to play ball when they were kids. He added that they used to call Mardig *The Kid*. Even though this was not true, I wanted to believe they knew each other. It was nice to know he believed they shared something in common. As confused as people's minds get with this disease, any bit of familiarity, whether real or imagined, comforts them.

We continued watching Mardig slowly eat his dinner. He reached for the white bread on his tray. His left hand shook a little as he brought the sandwich closer. He carefully wedged his right index finger in between the slices to see what was inside, pulled his finger out, and then took a big bite out of the soft buttered bread.

I couldn't get beyond the way my father looked sitting there, hunched over, his extended hand shaking slightly as he carefully grasped a spoonful of food and slowly brought it toward his mouth. We sat watching him, occasionally chatting, but mostly watching him.

"Doesn't he look cute?" I asked David after I watched my father for a long minute.

"Uhh, I suppose so," he replied.

I had not often referred to my father as cute. Yet there was something cute about him. He had this slightly helpless quality. After all, what would he do if this nice meal were not prepared for him? He couldn't fend for himself anymore. I sat there, thankful that he received such well-balanced meals and that he was still able to eat them. Someday he will have to be helped because he won't know how to feed himself. This is what happens to many people with Alzheimer's. It's only a matter of time.

There he was, hunched over, his mouth barely clearing the height of the dishes on his tray. He had to raise his elbow almost shoulder height to clear the tray when reaching for his food. With trembling hands, he carefully reached out and spooned or forked whatever he wanted. He liked soft food best—mashed potatoes, soft white bread, or stuffing. Sweet foods that were soft were even better!

David and I quietly watched him eat. Occasionally we looked around to the other residents and at the aides who were removing trays of food left by the residents.

When he was finished, Mardig reached over for a napkin and carefully wiped his mouth. He neatly folded his napkin and placed it on his tray. I handed him a toothpick—something he always liked to use after a meal. Toothpicks were considered *contraband* in the facility since residents could get poked by a misplaced toothpick. He glanced at me when I handed him the toothpick. He took it and used it briefly and then placed it toward the back of his tray. He stood up, picked up his tray, and handed it to the aide who smiled and thanked him. She looked over to us and said, "Martin always does this," meaning, he picks up his tray and brings it to the aides.

He then turned to us and said as politely as he could muster, "Well, it was my pleasure to join you for dinner. Thank you." Then he turned around and walked away. He quickly walked toward the doors to leave the dining room.

I sat there aghast. I was truly surprised at what had happened. My father had no clue who we were. And then David and I began to laugh. *What else could we do in a situation like this? It was truly comical. My father had no idea.*

∽   ∽

WHEN MARDIG FIRST CAME TO THE FACILITY, he'd worry about money. "I don't want to eat. Who's going to pay for it?"

"It's already paid for," we'd say.

"Who's paying for it?" he'd ask, genuinely curious about who was paying his way.

Sometimes, we'd say, "We are."

He didn't want to burden us and always responded, "I'll pay you back."

We said it was all right. It was really Mardig who was paying for everything. But because he didn't believe he had enough money, we didn't want him to worry. David and I talked about this and decided to change our reply in the future if he asked.

"The government is paying for all of this," we said the next time.

"It is? Why is the government paying for me?"

"Because you're retired and this is the benefit they provide." *What does one say? Sure it's a lie. But with his memory impaired, isn't it important to make him feel comfortable?*

"Good," he said happily.

He'd sometimes ask us for a dollar. Other times, he'd ask, "Do you have any money on you?"

"Yes," I'd reply.

"Can I have some?"

"How much?" I'd ask.

"How much have you got?"

I'd open my wallet and show him the twenties and tens inside. He'd grab a ten and say, "Thanks. This'll last me for a while. I'll pay you back," he'd add. Then he'd stuff the money into his left front pocket. As the months passed, he'd ask for less money—mostly change.

~   ~

AS MY FATHER'S CONDITION WORSENED, he would ask about Ma and Pop. Sometimes Ma was his mother, and other times she was his wife (my mother). We were unclear because he'd just ask, "Are you going to see Ma?" "How's Ma doing?" "How's Pop doing?"

Months earlier, we tried being truthful with him on all things. We'd remind him that his parents were long gone. This would depress him. He wouldn't know what to make of the information that his wife or his parents were no longer around. Sometimes, David used logic. He asked my father how old he was. Mardig used to guess he was in his seventies or eighties. David would add that his parents would have to be near one hundred if they were still alive. All of us would laugh, knowing how impossible such longevity was for our family. Then Mardig would change the subject.

The next time we'd visit, he asked the same questions. So, one day, during a support group meeting I raised the issue of honesty. After the meeting was over, Jeanne, one of the attendees who is caring for her mother, pulled me aside and asked me to consider something. She explained that given my father's forgetfulness, each time I told him his parents and wife were gone, I was making him relive the loss over again. She said, if I had a hard time lying, to just deflect the comment and to share pleasant memories of the person he's asking about. I thanked her and said I would give it a try.

The next time Mardig talked about Ma, my mother, I asked him if he remembered how we used to pack picnics for brunch at the lakefront on Sundays. He smiled and said he didn't remember but was amazed I did. He added, "You really enjoyed those, didn't you?" I nodded my head. It worked!

I couldn't thank Jeanne enough. It's hard because we wanted to be truthful. Yet, by being truthful we sometimes hurt an impaired person.

The question still remains, When do we tell the truth, and when don't we?

∿   ∿

WHILE I CONTINUED PROCESSING THE THINGS I brought from Mardig's house in Milwaukee, I thought about all the notes he took, the journals he kept so that he'd remember. In some journals he even wrote, "I'm writing this so I don't forget." Even while he lived with us, he'd take notes to make sense of his world. Sometimes, I saw it as a desperate measure to hang onto reality.

The things that really made me smile were his methodical qualities. As I was cleaning the closet of his room (in our house), I ran across some Halloween decorations. One was a three-foot coiled rubber snake. He had taken some packing thread and tightly wrapped the snake so it wouldn't uncoil. He even took pains to tie a half bow so that one could pull one end of the thread to easily untie his handiwork.

Seeing this took me back to Milwaukee. While cleaning out his desk and trying to quickly screen the important things from the unimportant, I found something unusual. Tape from an audiocassette was hand wrapped around an empty orange-colored spool of correcto-ribbon for electric typewriters. *What was his plan for this? Why would he take time to carefully hand wrap magnetic tape in this fashion?*

Everything had to be wrapped, boxed, and put away. And he'd always say, "I'll look at it later."

⌣ ⌣

IN OUR DAY-TO-DAY LIVES, small moments sneak by, barely noticed because they don't seem significant at the time. It's hard to know what to keep and what not to as I go through my father's things. I try not to throw away too much, even though I don't like collecting things.

I have a twenty-gallon container of sentimental things. However, I believe when we accumulate a lot we become slaves to our possessions. Each of my parents provided an example. It's an ongoing struggle. How do I know today what will have meaning for me tomorrow? I may experience something different in my life that will give me another angle of insight into my father.

Sorting through all his paperwork, much of it that may have been tossed as trash, yielded the following discoveries.

I noticed Mardig went through a phase in his thirties when he signed his name, *M. Avadian*—the initial of his first name and then his last name. Coincidentally, nearly a decade ago, I made the conscious decision to sign my name in the same way. The increasing amount of paperwork I had to sign made this a necessity. I experienced great pain in my wrist, and reasoned, if I had less to write, my wrist would not hurt as much. What a surprise when I saw that Mardig also abbreviated his first name when he was my age. In his forties, he went back to signing his complete name. I wonder if I'll do the same.

Mardig was a logical and rational man. He was a meticulous record keeper and I am pleased to hold his record books. He saved the receipts of my birth. It cost $150 to bring me into this world in 1959. He recorded when I had chicken pox. Perhaps the accompanying 106° fever damaged nerves which resulted in my inability to hear out of my left ear.

In his later years, Mardig tried to make sense of his finances and kept journals of letters he wrote to various banks, the IRS, and to attorneys in an attempt to collect money owed to him. This detailed record keeping started when he was much younger. Records showed that he followed a conservative and low-risk approach to his investments. Opting for U.S. Savings Bonds, CDs, and Treasury Funds, he rebuffed my suggestion in the mid-1980s to invest in the stock and options markets. Yet, in his earlier years, he bought stock in a number of companies. I'm not certain of the outcome of these early investments.

The *coup* came when I ran across an old document entitled, Fitch Stock Summary, April 1943 issue, by Harris, Upham, & Company. This summary contained stock prices during the years of the Great Depression. Surprisingly, AT&T's prices ranged from a high of $310.25 to a low of $70.25 from 1929 to 1942. GE's range was equally surprising, $100.75 to $8.50! IBM, $255 to $52.50! Accounting for all the stock splits that followed in the more than fifty years since then, I can't imagine what these stocks would be worth today. Commodities were also listed in this summary. No precious metals were traded at this time. But black pepper was a listed commodity in 1942! What a treasure!

These are the small moments that I cherish as I think about my father. After all, it's the little things that make lasting memories.

Epilogue

As of this writing, Mardig continues to thrive in the skilled nursing facility.

We celebrated his eighty-eighth birthday in August. He is not on any medications as of this writing and he's keeping his weight steady, between 118 and 120 pounds. He has slowed down noticeably and is more confused, but he still flirts with the aides.

He no longer recognizes David and me. When we visit him, he'll walk past us. When we say this to others, they say how hard this must be for us. I can't explain it, but it's not. We try to accept Mardig as he is. Sure, we would prefer that he recognized us and called us by name, as he did one afternoon in a sudden surge of awareness. As he was walking away from us, he abruptly turned, looked at me, and asked, "Hey, Brenda, who was that person who was going to take care of…?" I was astonished, because for three months prior, he had no idea who I was, much less that I was even a female. And in this one moment, he named me and knew I was his daughter!

Most of the time we can't have a conversation with him that makes sense. We ask about his day, his children, his wife, and his work at GE. He responds about something else—fixing the car, waiting for imaginary people. He even asks if we saw Ma and Pa (his parents) that day.

I am happy he is with us on this earth. I didn't think he'd live beyond March 1998. But he did. At this rate, I believe he'll greet the year 2000. It is far better for me to enjoy him with whatever his mind has to offer, than not to have him at all. He is not ready to die yet, and I am not ready to see him go. When this time comes, it will be our next challenge.

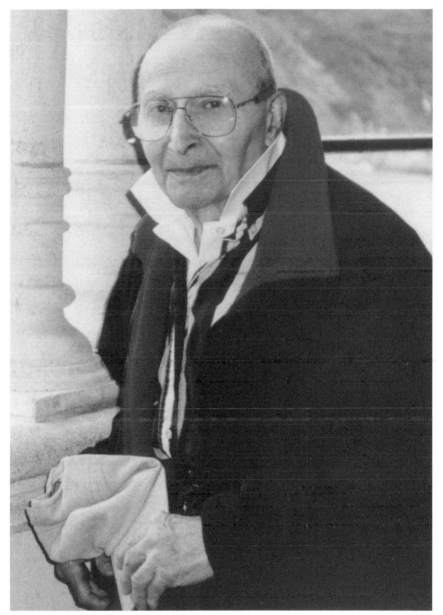

Martin Avadian at Catalina Island, March 1997.

Ten Suggestions for Caregivers

1. Break tasks down into single steps.

2. Meet people with Alzheimer's at the level/mood they are currently in.

3. Make direct eye contact when speaking.

4. Answer questions that are constantly repeated as if each was the first time it was asked.

5. No matter how bizarre their actions or how much they insult you, remember, especially in the later stages, they are no longer responsible for their actions and words.

6. It's okay to get frustrated and even angry. Be sure to find an appropriate outlet for your feelings—e.g., walking, calling a friend.

7. Seek support/help from others. Go to support group meetings regularly. Others are experiencing the same things you are (guilt, anxiety, frustration, uncertainty, depression, helplessness). Call your local Alzheimer's Association chapter for information on support group meetings in your area. If no support groups are available, consider starting one.

8. Take care of yourself. Get some rest. Set your boundaries around what you can manage. Don't be a martyr! (This is easier said than done.) If you are not well, you can't care for

another. Consider your options—adult day care, in-home care, board and care, nursing facility.

9. Smile and give a hug and kiss, if appropriate.

10. Seek appropriate professional advice, e.g., legal, financial, healthcare.

FOR MORE INFORMATION . . .

Alzheimer's Association
919 North Michigan Avenue, Ste. 1000
Chicago, IL 60611
312-335-8700
800-272-3900
http://www.alz.org

Agency for Health Care Policy and Research
Publications Clearing House
P.O. Box 8547
Silver Spring, MD 20907
800-358-9295

BIBLIOGRAPHY

Bell, Virginia and Troxel, David. *The Best Friends Approach to Alzheimer's Care*. Baltimore, MD: Health Professionals Press, 1996.

Davidson, Ann. *Alzheimer's, a Love Story: One Year in My Husband's Journey*. Seacaucus, NJ: Birch Lane Press, 1997.

Dyer, Joyce. *In a Tangled Wood: An Alzheimer's Journey*. Dallas, TX: Southern Methodist University Press, 1996.

Grollman, Earl A. and Kosik, Kenneth S. *When Someone You Love Has Alzheimer's: The Caregiver's Journey*. Boston, MA: Beacon Press, 1997.

Gruetzner, Howard. *Alzheimer's: A Caregiver's Guide and Sourcebook*. New York, NY: John Wiley & Sons, 1992.

Haisman, Pam. *Alzheimer's Disease: Caregiver's Speak Out*. Ft. Myers, FL: Chippendale House Publishers, 1998.

Howes, Zabbia, Kim. *Painted Diaries: A Mother and Daughter's Experience Through Alzheimer's*. Minneapolis, MN: Fairview Press, 1996.

Mace, Nancy L. and Rabins, Peter V. *The 36-Hour Day: A Family Guide to Caring for Persons with Alzheimer's Disease, Related Dementing Illness and Memory Loss in Later Life*. New York, NY: Warner Books, 1991.

Sarnoff, Schiff, Harriet. *How Did I Become My Parent's Parent?* New York, NY: Viking Press, 1996.

Strecker, Teresa R. Alzheimer's: *Making Sense of Suffering*. Lafayette, LA: Vital Issues Press, 1997.

Warren, Tom. *Beating Alzheimer's: A Step Towards Unlocking the Mysteries of Brain Diseases*. Garden City Park, NY: Avery Publishing Group, 1991.

Wexler, Nancy. *Mama Can't Remember Anymore: Care Management of Aging Parents and Loved Ones*. Thousand Oaks, CA: Wein & Wein Publishers, 1997.

INDEX

ORDER INFORMATION

If you are unable to obtain *"Where's my shoes?"* (ISBN: 0-9632752-1-6) from your local bookstore or the Internet, please send a check or money order, payable to:

North Star Books
P.O. Box 259
Lancaster, CA 93584-0259

Individuals and organizations wanting to order ten or more copies, please call toll free 1-888-349-1789 (voice mail only) for volume discount information.

Prices:
$21.95 each plus $3.75 for *Priority S&H* (for the first book, plus $1.50 for each additional book sent to the same address.)
California residents please add sales tax.
(Multiply book price total by .0825.)

If you would like to contact the author, you may write to her at the above address or send an e-mail to NSB@aol.com